WALDY, MYELO, & ME

WALDY, MYELO, & ME

SURVIVING WALDENSTRÖM'S MACROGLOBULINEMIA & MYELODYSPLASTIC SYNDROME

CAROL TURNER, MD

Advantage | Books

Published by Advantage, Charleston, South Carolina.
Member of Advantage Media.

ADVANTAGE is a registered trademark, and the Advantage colophon is a trademark of Advantage Media Group, Inc.

Printed in the United States of America.

10 9 8 7 6 5 4 3 2 1

ISBN: 978-1-64225-797-7 (Hardcover)
ISBN: 978-1-64225-796-0 (eBook)

Library of Congress Control Number: 2023905574

Cover design by Analisa Smith.
Layout design by Lance Buckley.

This publication is designed to provide accurate and authoritative information in regard to the subject matter covered. It is sold with the understanding that the publisher is not engaged in rendering legal, accounting, or other professional services. If legal advice or other expert assistance is required, the services of a competent professional person should be sought.

Advantage Media helps busy entrepreneurs, CEOs, and leaders write and publish a book to grow their business and become the authority in their field. Advantage authors comprise an exclusive community of industry professionals, idea-makers, and thought leaders. Do you have a book idea or manuscript for consideration? We would love to hear from you at **AdvantageMedia.com**.

To those affected by bone marrow and blood cancers

CONTENTS

PART I
MY BIG
MOLECULE

THE CALL

I am standing at a gas station in Gunnison, Colorado. My eighteen-year-old son and I are traveling to Durango to watch my two other sons compete in the Colorado State High School Mountain Bike Championship when the call comes through. I answer away from the car while he pumps the gas just in case it's bad news.

"You have a lymphoproliferative disorder," says the hematologist.

I am a pediatrician. I know what this means. This is a malignancy. Some prefer to call it "cancer."

The doctor says it looks like non-Hodgkin's lymphoma. He says we can do a bone marrow biopsy; a CT scan of my chest, abdomen, and pelvis; or both. I vote for both. The doctor tells me he hopes that it's not aggressive, then hangs up.

This phone call plunges me into an abyss of worry, loss of control, imagined worst-case scenarios, questions with no answers, grief, and sadness. This definitely counts as bad news.

I am about to give an Academy Award–worthy performance in betraying nothing of my shock or crushing emotional pain to my son. He's a freshman in college and needs to study. He does *not* need to worry about his mom having cancer. He has no clue I'm even sick. I certainly don't look sick.

My son drives. We make our way through Ouray and over Red Mountain Pass toward Silverton. It is spectacular, one of my favorite drives in the entire state—dramatic, awe-inspiring beauty at every turn.

Whenever we have a cell signal, I google non-Hodgkin's lymphoma. This is a terrible idea. Everything looks horrendous. I read about one-year remission rates, five-year survival rates, scores for risk, endless drugs, and options for treatment plans.

How do they even begin to figure out a treatment plan? Do they plug in my age, symptoms, blood test results, and bone marrow and scan results, and some machine spits out my chemo formula? Is there an app for this?

Though I know I shouldn't, I keep reading and reading. All of the credible sites weigh in: Cedars-Sinai, Mayo Clinic, American Cancer Society, Dana-Farber. All fail miserably in telling me what I want to hear: that there is a cure and that I will be cured. I do not want to hear any euphemistic cancer lingo from my doctor: remission, five-year survival, treatment options, promising clinical trial. I want to hear the word "cure."

I tell my husband when we get to Durango. He's already in bed and asks me an innocent question about taking a short hike the next day. I immediately start sobbing and reply that no, I cannot go on a short hike because I have cancer.

He knows that I've been undergoing tests and tells me we'll do what we need to do to beat it. I tell him I'm worried about losing my hair. He tells me that that's the least of our worries.

As if. I love my hair. I want to look nice. I don't want to look haggard and sickly. I want to look fit and healthy. There is a certain amount of vanity in my personal concerns, especially now that I feel damaged, diseased, and gross.

For the next two days, I try not to inflict myself upon others. I do not want to tell my kids. They don't need this. They are here this weekend to race mountain bikes for twenty-four miles.

THE PAIN

And when it's raining
Raining hard
That's when the rain will
Break my heart
Raining, raining
In the heart

—U2, "ONE TREE HILL"

I awaken to walk the dogs, as I do first thing every morning. I love the city of Durango. I love bike races. I love doing things outdoors with my family. And I loved mornings. But now mornings are the worst. *This* morning my first thought is, *I have cancer.*

I need to write a will. I need to close my solo rural pediatric practice. I need to call the crematorium, and my husband needs to start dating.

I am not who I was less than twenty-four hours ago. That person is gone. I sob for the first couple of hours of the morning, sitting alone in the truck. Wailing, moaning, thrashing, bawling. Floods of tears. By midmorning I have cried as much as I can. Eventually, it gets boring.

I go up to watch the races, support the team, see my kids, and avoid my friends. I don't want to tell them a thing. They *used* to think I was awesome; now I'm a cancer patient. It's already defining me. My husband suggests that it's not healthy to wallow so much. I respond with my typical scorched-earth emotional overreaction: everything's fine, and I know that he's happy I'm dying.

After the races, my youngest son drives us back home by a different route. The song "Cancer" by Twenty One Pilots randomly plays from his Spotify. Obviously, it's all part of the greater conspiracy. I hide my sobbing over Wolf Creek Pass. As we drive by the Sangre de Cristo Mountains, I look out the window at Little Bear and Blanca Peaks, Crestone Peak, and Crestone Needle. I have climbed them all.

These mountains are among the most challenging, dangerous, and rewarding in all of Colorado. Summiting these fourteen-thousand-foot peaks, otherwise known as "the fourteeners," is among the greatest accomplishments of my life. I have climbed all except one: Culebra Peak.

I'm glad I get to see these mountains again, here in the final thirty-six hours of my life. The more I think about my cancer, the shorter my anticipated life span becomes. In fact, I'm not sure I will survive the five-hour drive home.

The next morning I walk the dogs, make breakfast for the kids, do the laundry, clean the kitchen, and get ready for work, all as usual. When I get in the car and start to put on my seat belt, I ponder the stupid futility of doing so.

Why am I putting on this dumb seat belt? What are the chances I'm going to get in a car accident in the three-mile drive to school versus getting cancer? Oh. Wait. I *do* have cancer. There's a 100 percent chance of that. Looking at it statistically, there is no reason to wear the seat belt. I'm already toast.

THE LIFE REVIEW

My decision to go into pediatrics was heavily influenced by a child I saw as a medical student in the mideighties. We'd just had our leukemia lecture as part of our pediatrics rotation, and immediately afterward, in the clinic, I picked up the next chart in the rack before walking in to see my patients.

This six-year-old girl had fevers, fatigue, gum bleeding, bruising, leg pain, and weight loss. The more she talked, the more I knew that she had acute lymphocytic leukemia, the most common pediatric blood cancer. She bravely listed her painful and scary symptoms without whining or complaining, oblivious to the dreaded diagnosis to come.

This moment crystallized a sequence of events that would in so many ways come to shape my life: absorbing information; combining it with my knowledge; applying it to the case of a living, breathing person; and impacting, if not always saving, a child's life. She was treated and survived to remission, and that's the last I knew of her.

I practiced pediatric emergency medicine for ten years, then hung my own shingle and opened a solo rural practice in the foothills outside of Denver. While my family is my proudest accomplishment—my husband in particular loves being categorized as an "accomplishment"—my career is a close second. I feel fortunate to love my job every single day. I love walking into my office, I love my employees, and I love taking care of the infants, children, teens, and young adults who come to see me.

Coming in at a very close third are my various milestones in competitive and recreational sports. My husband and I share a deep mutual love of recreation in Colorado. For years we were avid rock climbers, whitewater kayakers, backpackers, hikers, "fourteenerers," skiers, and mountain bikers and have shared these passions with our sons.

Aside from a little hiatus for pregnancies and then raising young kids, I've always sought out amateur sports competitions. I completed a full-distance, off-road XTERRA Triathlon and a local half-triathlon when my youngest son was around five. I was slow, but I finished both.

After that, I started in on mountain bike races and bicycle motocross (BMX) because our sons were competing in these events. BMX is crazy fun, and it took hold of me. I've been racing BMX for seven years, and I didn't even start until fifty. In mountain biking, I love the scenery, slowly grinding up the hills, then screaming back down them. My screaming down is not objectively very high velocity, but it feels fast to me. I compete in the old lady categories, and my kids are not impressed. I love a flowy, smooth, winding trail, with mom-sized obstacles on the downhill.

This past summer my legs hurt more than they usually did at the end of BMX races. Recovery was harder. I'm "old," but I never once thought I was sick. Endurance mountain bike rides and races were the biggest problems. I had to stop and turn back on approaches before even getting to steep ascents I'd routinely conquered the season prior. My first thoughts were, *Maybe I need to train more. And train harder. Maybe I have a little bug. Maybe I'm having a bad day. Maybe I'm a little tired.*

There was a tangible difference from the prior summer to the most recent. In the previous season, I could power up steep hills at altitude and felt great. Then gradually I had to get off the bike and sit down to recover my aching legs and bring down my heart rate. I was immediately fatigued by muscle pain, as if I'd been riding for many miles at a fast pace. Suddenly, I was finding myself remarkably, debilitatingly short of breath.

After ignoring and brushing off these symptoms, I entered a mountain bike race with my oldest son and had to repeatedly get off the bike, sit down in the dirt, and recover before pedaling a few more strokes. I could not force myself to power up the hills. I ultimately finished the race but knew something was wrong. It was not "just a bad day" or a bug. I had trained. I was sick.

The crippling shortness of breath was beyond a fitness issue; it was pathologic. Had I not been so deeply involved in sports, I probably wouldn't have noticed that anything was wrong. At that time, walking, daily living, and working were no problem, but biking uphill hurtled me into a sick, deep canyon of ache. Biking was my sentinel event. It gave me the foundational clue.

THE DOCTORS

After busting through the denial, I accepted that it was not just a little bug or merely needing to train more. I was sick—really sick. I went to see a whole mess of doctors. I saw a gastroenterologist, cardiologist, and gynecologist. I was diagnosed with anemia—the condition of having too few oxygen-rich red blood cells, which makes you feel tired. Anemia is measured as a low hemoglobin, and my hemoglobin was very low. We could not find the cause, and it didn't respond to common treatment.

It was supposed to be an easy fix. At that point it became clear that there was something more seriously wrong. I knew that cancer was a possibility, but I can't say that I considered it a *realistic* one. I'm healthy, except for being sick.

I go to the hematologist. There, I'm delighted to be shown to the exam room in the hallway marked with a sign that reads, "Benign Hematology." Good. Exactly where I belong!

Passing through oncology, I take in all the incredibly sick cancer patients and feel so sad for them. Some are clearly at late stages in their disease. There are some in wheelchairs and others who need assistance to walk. Most are thin and weak, with skin of a greenish-bronze-yellow color. They're on their way, variously, to the radiation oncology unit, the bone marrow transplant unit, or the clinical trials unit. I am selfishly glad I am not one of the cancer patients—these poor, unfortunate *other people*.

My hematologist, Dr. Blood Expert, sees something subtle in my blood cell counts and chemistry. It makes him suspicious of an abnormal cell line and, more specifically, an abnormal protein-producing line. I do not understand or know exactly what clues him in; after all, he's the expert. He tells me we're going to do an entire workup.

I had walked into this office hoping to be taken seriously regarding my anemia and, more importantly, my inability to ride a mountain bike up a steep hill at nine thousand feet at fifty-seven years of age. I was anxious that they might brush off my concerns and tell me to take up a more age-appropriate pastime, such as knitting.

I should have known better. This is Colorado. We're an active state. No one downplays my symptoms. Dr. Blood Expert immediately saw my passions, believed my symptoms, saw a blood disorder, and directed my care with the highest level of concern.

In his office I could tell he thought it might be bad. He had the look of maintaining professionalism and the right dose of honesty but hesitated to spill all the beans before his suspicions were confirmed.

Which brings us back to that drive to Durango, the phone call, and the first time anyone verbalized that I had it.

Cancer. Lymphoma. *Non-Hodgkin's* lymphoma.

THE BONE MARROW BIOPSY

Shout

Shout

Let it all out

These are the things I can do without

—TEARS FOR FEARS, "SHOUT"

D r. Blood Expert tells me that my choices are to get the bone marrow biopsy done right away, without sedation, or to wait a few weeks for a sedation spot. No question there: I want this done. Yesterday. No sedation it is.

Now for a brief review of all the things about which I am pissy. I am pissy about the parking lot at the cancer center. It requires an inconvenient left turn, and it is hard to find a spot big enough for my truck. I am pissy that I'm about to need an oncologist. Just *saying* "oncologist" makes me fussy. This is not so much a personal, specific mad; it's more global, revolving around the fact that cancer exists in the first place. I hate that I have to come here and that I am now officially a cancer patient.

The staff at the center are all professional, positive, caring, and efficient, which also really pisses me off. I want to scream at each and every one of them. I'm not feeling positive, polite, or engaging or particularly receptive to their caring natures. As everyone continues to look terribly sick in the waiting room, the nurses have their extra-nurturing faces on. These are nice people, and I want nothing to do with any of them. I hate this place.

Soon the phlebotomist is about to cry; she has to stick me three times before she gets any of my blood. I don't care. I get it. I've done loads of blood draws. I reassure her that I'm fine and that I understand that these things don't always go as planned.

I want to ride my bike. I want to walk the dogs without feeling exhausted. This dumb anemia has left me with zero exercise tolerance. Now merely walking up a flight of stairs is taxing. I haven't exercised in two months, which also makes me *just* a bit grumpy.

To my knowledge, my kids haven't noticed anything wrong. I still do the same things at home, and I'm not missing any work. Work is vital. A few friends, however, are a bit too perceptive, and they're beginning to show oppressive concern. I haven't been at the BMX track or on the mountain bike trails, and they notice. My calendar used to have entries like "bike practice," "bike race," "son's lacrosse game." Now it says "CT scan," "bone marrow biopsy," "lab draw."

At this point, only my husband knows, and I'm maintaining secrecy for the time being. I'm not ready for anyone else to know. I need more information, and I am *definitely* not ready for my kids to know.

Now for the bone marrow biopsy. Quite frankly I'm petrified as I deal with the cheery and helpful parking attendant who found a spot for my truck, the excessively positive front desk check-in lady, the kind preprocedure phlebotomist, and the preposterously perky medical assistant who guides me to the death chamber procedure room.

The experienced nurse practitioner who will be performing the torture explains that she will use a power drill to enter the bone and that there will be a local anesthetic to numb it. She says it looks and sounds just like any other power drill, and then she holds up the drill and makes the *whirrr* noise. I'm going to barf.

13

I'm lying facedown as they prepare to drill into my pelvis and suck out marrow. The nurse practitioner explains that because the marrow compartment is finite, the biopsy can cause a jolt as pressure enters a closed space. Super.

I feel dizzy, weak, and nauseated, but I'm also determined to get this done. I've not only seen these but also even performed them in training but using what's called a *trocar* instead of a drill. The visual is making it worse. This is already painful, and she hasn't even started.

Soon the local anesthetic is in, and the drill is whirring.

"There we go! I've popped into the bone. We're just sucking out the marrow. Now for the biopsy."

The biopsy feels like a hot skewer attached to an air compressor, propelled by a train, which is inflating a tire in my pelvic bone. Deep, agonizing pain radiates down my leg, through the table, into the floor, and back up to my spine. I have never felt such a chilling pain.

"Okay! And we're all done!" says Nurse Ratchet. If I do this again, next time I'm getting the sedation—one milligram below the toxic dose.

The CT scans of my chest, abdomen, and pelvis are normal. There is no mass, the cancer has not spread to my lymph nodes, and my coronary arteries look completely clear! But for now I do not have a specific diagnosis; I'll have to wait another two weeks for that. For now it's just garden-variety "cancer." In my bone marrow, something's amiss.

THE WAIT

How do I tell my kids? Clearly I've been tired. I haven't been able to do much of anything. They may have noticed, but I'm not entirely sure.

I decide to tell my two younger sons when they get into the car after school. I tell them I have been seeing doctors and undergoing tests, have cancer in my bone marrow, am getting the best possible care, and will fight this with everything that I have.

Then I repeat, "Yes, I have cancer."

They do not say anything on the drive home. I remain quiet. This is a lot for them to process.

Later, when I see him, I tell my oldest son. Guess what. He already knew! He heard me tell my husband the very first night in Durango. We were in the same hotel room. I thought he was asleep.

All along he was waiting for me to be ready to talk about it. He knew that I wanted to avoid him being worried and distracted. Now *that's* a nice kid.

I work, shop, clean, cook, and take care of the house and look wistfully at my bikes—all noble uses of one's time. I try to be there for my family as much as I can be, but I'm

> I'm determined to not let this diagnosis take over our family's day-to-day functioning, even as it's taken over my body.

weak, emotional, and worried. I check my email and phone every minute, awaiting the next test result. I sleep a ton, and am generally in bed even more. My husband, sons, dogs, and the cat all come to sit with me in the afternoons and evenings for family conversations. It's kind of sweet.

I'm determined to not let this diagnosis take over our family's day-to-day functioning, even as it's taken over my body. If you hadn't noticed, one of my primary goals is to minimize the negative impact of my cancer on my kids. My husband will be fine. He's solid as a rock.

Each day is different. There are good days and bad days. All the while, I'm a walking cliché of chronic disease catchphrases. Some days I feel pretty good and try to get more done. Others, I'm exhausted and can't wait to sit down. Sometimes I feel winded simply talking to my patients. By midafternoon, I'm absolutely cooked and go straight to bed when I get home. I'll do a load of laundry after taking a nap, then I have to lie right back down. What a weird way to function.

The cancer has not yet eaten me up; after all, here I am, writing about it. I'd love to have definitive treatment to fix the anemia, and it would be great to have the energy to wash the dishes and talk at the same time.

When I email Dr. Blood Expert through the patient portal, he tells me not to write my own obituary just yet. How did he know? He also advised me to forget everything I learned in medical school about cancer, staging, and survival. None of it means anything anymore. Everything has changed: definitions, research, technology, treatments, data, understanding, and survival rates; all continue to progress at a lightning pace.

Now that I may live and have the free time, I should probably also cancel my reservation at the crematorium and tell my husband to shut down his dating sites.

I'm sitting in front of a fire in a coffee shop in Keystone as I write this. Up on the mountain, my middle son and two of his friends are skiing. I feel cancer-sick. You have to have cancer to know this feeling; it's a combination of aches, chills, fatigue, more aches, misery, and general yuck.

I am not skiing. I do not even *consider* skiing. Mentally this is a continental shift. I can feel myself slipping back into being a sad, weak mess. I'm smashing into the cancer-reality wall, still trying to protect my kids from their mom as an emotional disaster.

THE DIAGNOSIS

We were so close, there was no room
We bled inside each other's wounds
We all had caught the same disease

−MELANIE SAFKA, "LAY DOWN (CANDLES IN THE RAIN)"

We have bone marrow results: Waldenström's lymphoma. It has a few other catchy monikers: lymphoplasmacytic lymphoma, Waldenström's macroglobulinemia. Macroglobulinemia is a fancy word for a big, annoying, fat, stupid protein molecule in the blood. Waldenström's lymphoma. Why does it have such a stupid cancer name? Can't they call it Supercross lymphoma? Mogul run lymphoma? BMX lymphoma?

Guess where I get to go again now. Back to the lab for more blood work! It's hard to believe that there are still tests they've not yet run on me. Back to the dreaded parking lot and my new exercise routine: walking into the clinic, back to the waiting room, and on to the lab.

This time it's crowded. Again, everyone looks so sad and sick. New cancer patients in the same palette of colors: orange, bronze, green, pale yellow. We're all on different schedules, so I'll never know how any of the others ultimately fare in fighting their own battles. Though we all have this monstrous thing in common, we do not interact. Cancer is a great equalizer and great insulator. Our malignant cells do not care about us as human beings. They want to live, which means that we may die. We're all essentially the same here in this waiting room: cancer cell vessels.

In the grocery store, dentist's office, post office, or dry cleaners, when they ask if you're having a nice day, there's at least a chance that you are. When you're checking in at the cancer center and they ask the same question, there's absolutely no chance. Not a single patient here is having a nice day. Not the twentysomething lady in the headscarf, not the elderly gentleman in his wheelchair, and certainly not me. All of us, without question, are having a sucky day.

The phlebotomist asks me if I've been hydrating. Oh yes, I'm the poster child of hydration. I've had two liters of water, one liter of sports drink, and two cups of chicken broth.

Three pokes for the blood draw. Again, they thank me for not being mad. Oh, I *am* mad, just not at *them*. I'm mad at this loser, Waldenström, who had to invent this dumb cancer. Everyone knows Walden Pond and Waldenbooks. But Walden*ström*? I endearingly name my cancer Waldy.

I sort of foggily remember it from the deepest recesses of medical school. There are 1,500 cases of Waldenström's in the United States per year, which makes it very, very rare. It's probably a genetic mutation, but no one knows for sure.

I googled my new life expectancy: five to twenty-five years. At least that narrows it down a bit. The extent of treatment options is dizzying and overwhelming to even look at.

My hematologist, Dr. Blood Expert, thinks I'm closer to the twenty-five-year survival contingent than the five. He even says that I'll get back on my bike again, but I may not be as fast. Wrong answer, pal; if you do your job, I'll be *faster*.

I wait five days to meet my new oncologist—five brutal, gruesome days, plagued by a deteriorating emotional state, hopelessness, crying, and being generally convinced that there is no help for me. I'm weak, cold, and shivering all the while.

They tell me that my husband must come to help make decisions because I may not be in the best emotional place to objectively receive the information. They don't want my state to lead to "rushed decisions" or a "suboptimal thought process."

Whatever. These cancer staffers think they know so much. As if my husband, the architect, knows how to make decisions about my cancer.

Okay, fine. I guess he can come. C'mon, Waldy, we're all going to see the doctor.

The front desk lady gives me a form and explains that it's for all new cancer patients to log and assess their "life impact"—1 for least, 10 for most. Eye roll.

On the sheet of paper, there are four categories with a rating scale of 1 to 10. I dutifully fill it out. Emotional Impact: 10. Social Impact: 10. Health Impact: 10. Practical Impact: 10. I drip tears on each rating scale to enhance the effect.

My husband is not here yet. He probably found a bimbo on Tinder for cancer widowers needing extra affection.

Ah, here he comes now! No bimbo.

THE EDUCATION

My new doctor is a real know-it-all, just like his staff. Dr. Know-It-All draws a picture of the big molecule: immunoglobulin M or IgM. IgM is in excess in my body, and it's being produced at the expense of good molecules. He emphasizes that this is a big, fat, XXL, huge, ginormous protein molecule. My big, bad protein molecule is coming from the bad lymphoma cells, which are otherwise busy taking over the good cells in my bone marrow. He tells me it's perhaps manageable but not curable. What a pisser.

Waldy is an IgM factory. In a healthy state, IgM is a normal part of the immune system and an infection-fighting molecule. But my IgM is not normal. This big, fat protein is not fighting infection, and Waldy is cranking it out in excess.

On top of that, I have way, way too little of immunoglobulins A and G, which are desperately needed for infection-fighting. This explains why I've had two rounds of shingles within the space of a few months. Remarkably, I've managed to avoid any other significant infections or acute illnesses despite being a general pediatrician who's exposed to germs literally all the livelong day. I must be an even more fanatical hand-washer than I thought.

Dr. Know-It-All, who will hereafter receive additional honorifics depending on my mood, reviews three programs and combinations. One will be a combination of immunotherapy (biologic) infusions, chemotherapy injections, and high-dose steroids.

Sweet! Targeted chemo! I won't lose my hair! I'm calling to schedule with the salon as soon as I leave this dump.

My husband and I agree on the plan that Dr. Big-Shot Know-It-All recommends, which is on the aggressive side. We're comfortable that he can and will take care of me. I ask him if I can ride my bike again when I am better. He says yes and that he'll make me faster.

My husband tells Dr. Know-It-All that he has seen me tired. Indeed, he has seen me after telemark skiing in waist-deep powder in Alta, Utah, all day without stopping. He has seen me after climbing Mount Wilson and El Diente Peak, plus the connecting ridge. He has seen me through three pregnancies and three deliveries. He has seen me bike Monarch Crest, Colorado, thirty-five miles on a mountain bike. He has seen me hike Buckskin-Paria canyons in Utah and Arizona—thirty-eight miles when you factor in the bike ride to get there. But he has *never* seen me this tired.

> Cancer sucks, and you are going to feel like crap. Deal with it as well as you can. You may as well suck it up because you have no other choice.

So far my most profound advice is this: cancer sucks, and you are going to feel like crap. Deal with it as well as you can. You may as well suck it up because you have no other choice. Part of the process entails lots of waiting and an acceptance of the stepwise nature of diagnosis and treatment. Every cancer is different, and every patient is different. I learned to start trying to exchange *curable* for *treatable* and *manageable*. Find doctors that you trust. If possible, find a spouse you trust.

By the time I leave the center, everything on my impact form has gone down from a ten to a two; I never even turned it in. I even start to feel a measure of gratitude; I'm so grateful for cycling sports. On so many levels, I don't know where I'd be without them. I'm perhaps even more grateful for the scientists and cancer researchers who develop the modern therapies that treat common and rare malignancies. Mine is rare, yet I can get treatment.

Now the question is: Upon what do I focus my energy? I decide to be the best cancer patient they've ever had at that center. I will follow every instruction precisely. I will be on time, agreeable, cooperative, communicative, and sweet, though that last one will be a challenge. I will do what they tell me to do *exactly*. I will be tough through infusions and chemo. I will not complain. And as we annihilate this cancer, I want the front desk to star my chart with a "delightful patient" notation.

This is my newest amateur competitive event. I am going to pummel, trounce, suffocate, eradicate, trash, and thrash this cancer. Waldy, you are going down.

THE SECOND WAIT

I will start at 0700 hours in ten days. I will get labs drawn, and I will visit with my doctor, the oncology pharmacist, the dietitian, and the oncology social worker.

The staff feels that I may benefit from talking to the social worker for emotional and mental health support. They must have picked up on my precarious sanity. The scheduler wants to make sure I will accept this kind of help. Oh yes, I am all about this kind of help. I'm going to talk this lady's ear off. She will sit at my bedside until I am cheered the fuck up.

I love having a job to go to after I take the boys to school in the morning. Without it, I would probably wallow all day, ruminating, churning, and most likely becoming more paranoid about insurance companies plotting my demise. While seeing my own patients, I compartmentalize very well. The moms and dads and their newborns give me something to focus on. I particularly love four-year-olds, who have so much to say about life.

One comes in, and her father doesn't need to answer any questions because his kid has it covered. She tells me that she rides a two-wheel bike, wears her helmet every time, skis the blue runs, and is learning to swim. She likes her friends in preschool. Her favorite toys are airplanes and horses. She says she cannot draw a good person, but she can draw a velociraptor. Her sister bugs her, and her parents have never asked

24

her to do any chores. She knows the word "velociraptor" but does not know the word "chore." Sure, kid.

A nine-year-old boy comes in with his mother for his wellness visit. I ask him if he thinks he's getting enough exercise—a standard question. He says he thinks he does. He skis and says he recently competed in a ski enduro, which I ask him to explain. It was held at Arapahoe Basin Ski Area, he says. I know it well. It has one of the steepest inbound ski runs in North America, known as Pallavicini.

The kid goes on to tell me that the ski enduro is where competitors ski down Pallavicini as many times as possible in a full ski day. I'm thinking, *If this nine-year-old is tough, he could do eight to ten Pallavicini runs. That would be an epic day.*

I ask how many runs he completed in his ski enduro. Forty-three runs, he says.

Forty-three runs! He officially wins his age group. I'm going to say that the kid gets his exercise.

I love Colorado.

THE FIRST TREATMENT DAY

Watch the road and memorize
This life that pass before my eyes
And nothing is going my way

−R.E.M., "FIND THE RIVER"

It's zero dark thirty, and I'm driving into the clinic, pondering all the worthy reasons I've previously gotten on the road at such an ungodly hour: fourteeners, whitewater kayak paddling, ski days, backpacking, camping, mountain bike rides, climbing, rustic overnight hut trips. And lots of bike races and cycling events as both participant and spectator: enduros, dual slaloms, downhill and cross-country mountain bike races, fat bike races in the snow, BMX.

Every summer for forty-plus years, Estes Park, Colorado, "the YMCA of the Rockies," was our family trip. My dad took me to climb Longs Peak at age eight and then for many years thereafter. My dad is from Brooklyn. He knew nothing about any of this, but he still took his three young daughters up Longs Peak with the YMCA hiking program. It was a monumental, life-shaping event and one of the primary reasons I moved to Colorado: the love of summiting mountains. We'd meet our hiking group at 2:30 a.m. to drive to the trailhead. *That* was a solid reason to get up in the dark.

Today, however, I'm driving in the early morning, from dark to sunrise, with my molecule in tow. It's my first chemo trek, an off-road infusion adventure. I needed a new morning sport anyway. *Molecule destruction pursuit.* That's my sunrise sport, heading toward the Death Star.

As I walk under the Cancer Pavilion sign and into the building, reality hits me like a breaking wave. I've been thoroughly distracted by fear and sadness but had not quite gotten to *acceptance.*

Now truth and mortality have arrived: I am starting treatment for cancer.

The infusion center is a marvel, a bastion of expertise in highly specialized cancer treatment. Just one poke for my IV, then labs sent. My hemoglobin is down another point. There's a case conference to be held today with more supersmart blood disorder doctors. They're all here to review my bone marrow. Dr. Know-It-All, compulsive as usual, is worried we do not yet have the whole story. Oh great. How much more can there be?

Dexamethasone, a steroid, is the drug I'm given; it's the one that threatens to make the patient agitated and then crash. In it goes, and indeed, I feel quite agitated. Manic is another word that comes to mind. I cannot lie or sit still, I am continually moving my legs around in different positions, and my thoughts are racing. I'm ready to run laps around the parking lot. I feel as if I could push out the window and fly onto neighboring rooftops with my blanket for a cape. This lasts for about twenty minutes, then I calm down enough to receive the plethora of pre-infusion warnings and instructions.

Let me tell you about my nurse, who was placed on this earth to be an oncology infusion nurse. She is the epitome of competence inspiring confidence. Experienced, knowledgeable, caring, efficient, professional, and hardworking, she is nurse excellence personified. She anticipates, she listens, and she reacts.

She instructs me to tell her immediately if I have hives, itching, or throat tightening, but meanwhile, this infusion is going great.

They pretreat for allergic reactions, which are common with mouse gut infusions. You heard that right: my biologic infusion is a synthetic antibody that attaches to and explodes lymphoma cells, and it is made from *mice*.

The nurse keeps cranking up on the rate. I'm thinking, *This will be a breeze. I'll be out of here in a flash!*

Then, *Whoa. I* am *itching.*

I have red, raised hives, and my throat is tightening. I'm having difficulty swallowing and cannot take a deep breath.

I wonder if I should tell her.

While she did mention that this *is* something that would be important to tell her, I really want to push through and not be an alarmist. I delay and indulge in these irrational thought patterns for another minute, then finally tell her.

She exhibits no panic whatsoever, then springs into action. She stops the infusion to administer three more medications—two through the IV and one by mouth. The hives start to fade, and after two minutes, I can breathe. Brilliant.

We pause, restart at a slower rate, then repeat the circus act two more times. Three total episodes of allergic reactions: more difficulty breathing, throat-tightening, itching all over, hives. It lasts for eleven hours, but we get the infusion done.

Several visitors come by. My husband tries to take photos. Please, honey, no. I look green and dead.

Next, my social worker is an angelic gem. Sweet voice, soothing demeanor. She makes me aware of services available to me, then asks me about my cancer treatment goals. This is easy; I was prepared for harder questions. I want to minimize the negative impact of this illness on my kids, husband, patients, and employees. I want to continue performing my mom duties. I do not want to miss more work than

THE FIRST TREATMENT DAY

is necessary. I *need* to work. I want to manage my small business and care for my patients.

And of course, I want to get back to training and biking as soon as I feel well enough. My physical rehab plan is to join a gym to rebuild strength, commence spin training, and go to the climbing gym for tone and stretching. Then I'll get back on my BMX and mountain bikes to work back up to hard rides and competition. I also tell her that I want to keep writing this cancer tale and get it published.

> I want to minimize the negative impact of this illness on my kids, husband, patients, and employees.

Ms. Smooth-as-Silk Social Worker suggests that I am too intense, too type A. I need more balance. Unfortunately for her and her not-so-insightful commentary, I am not going through cancer treatment to change my personality. If I don't do the laundry, wash the dishes, and cook breakfast, I become obsolete. I will feel dead before I *am* dead. That's one of the big risks of cancer—it kills you before you die.

After she leaves, I suffer one of the most iconic degradations known to man—pushing my IV pole to the bathroom.

Well, that settles it—I am officially no longer cool.

THE GREAT NEWS

You're moving through the rough waters ...
This is now, this is here this is me ...
You're coming onto something so fast, so numb
That you can't even feel

—R.E.M., "SO FAST, SO NUMB"

Dr. Know-It-All returns. I am tired and groggy from the three rounds of allergy medications and my little loss of breath episodes, and it's my eleventh hour of infusion. This was a big day, and it's about to get a whole lot bigger. The pathologists have reviewed my bone marrow, and they believe that there's an additional abnormality there: the known lymphoma is taking up 40 percent of the marrow.

There are also too many large, immature, undifferentiated stem cells hanging around. If my marrow and stem cell system were functioning, they would mature, transform into red blood cells, make their way into my bloodstream, and then proceed to make themselves useful and exist in sufficient abundance to make me not anemic.

Instead, after getting bogged down and stuck, now they're just sitting in limbo, hanging out, and not turning into red blood cells. This condition is known as myelodysplasia, or myelodysplastic syndrome (MDS), which can become an aggressive leukemia at any time. It, too, is malignant.

With this condition, anemia is hard to treat: the red blood cells are slow to recover, some patients are transfusion dependent, and on top of everything else, the condition is indolent and slow-growing. If the MDS turns aggressive, I will need a bone marrow transplant.

So both of my cancers are indolent. Isn't that sweet of them?

Apparently, while I was being infused, there was a heated debate as to the best course of treatment for me. I feel so popular! Two "nerd" oncologists—"nerd" was the very word my oncologist used—are of the opinion that I should also be treated for myelodysplasia.

Dr. Know-It-All, living up to his name, stood firm. He believes that my symptoms are the result of the presence of the large lymphoma in my bone marrow and the IgM that it's producing. The IgM is causing increased blood viscosity, thick blood, and poor blood flow to my leg muscles and lungs. This certainly fits the symptom picture. He feels we should treat this aggressively, as we are, right then and there and *then* evaluate my response.

I am not processing this well. It's too much at once. He's obligated to tell me all of this, and I don't know what to say. Ultimately, I put my trust in his decisions. I could tell he'd thought about it, weighed the options, received input from other experts, and felt strongly about staying the course.

They'll need to perform a repeat bone marrow biopsy after my four months of treatment to assess my progress on the lymphoma, a.k.a. Waldy, then reassess the myelodysplasia, whom I christen Myelo.

After a top-off of chemo is injected into my arm, there's an additional superspecialist that I need to see. I ask where this guy is, thinking I may get sent to Boston or Houston. Nope, he's across the hall. How convenient!

After that, I drive myself home, though I should not be behind the wheel.

I have *two* cancers. Two cancers! Lymphoma *and* leukemia. Is this "Oh, by the way..." cancer worse than the original? In any case my bone marrow is seriously messed up. At least I trust the people taking care of me.

I'm going to have to be get comfortable with a lot of analyses in my near future. My team warned me that I'll feel very sick over the next couple of days and will have to push through. I'm so tired but glad to be done with my first treatment and finally going home. There's too much to ponder.

THE EFFECTS

The day after my first infusion bonanza, I feel great—the greatest I've felt in months. This steroid-blast euphoria lasts for a day.

Forty-eight hours after the infusion, the giddy feeling gives way to what I have termed the treatment *bonk*—a day of aches caused by the cancer cells inside of me dying en masse. The *technical* term is cell lysis, which refers to the malignant cells bursting and releasing their toxic contents, but *bonk* has a nicer ring to it.

Aches come in all flavors, but this sets a new bar for aching. Tumor cell lysis ache is deep, allover, all-encompassing. Every cell in my body—every part of every cell and every sub-particle of every cell—it all aches. My *mitochondria* ache.

My body feels as if it's decaying from the inside. Chills. Crushing fatigue. I'm dizzy, stumbly, weepy, and mopey. During the first night of posttreatment inferno, I am wondering how sick I'm *supposed* to feel. *Should* I feel this way? Is this a complication? Should I go to the hospital? Am I sick enough to call the cancer center nurse line? Is this expected? It's hard to tell.

I stay home, in bed, feeling like a corpse. Despite drinking liters of fluids, I have dry mouth and am light-headed and foggy. My vision is blurred. My aches are a ten on a one-to-ten scale. I don't know if the human body can truly withstand this assault. Everything hurts so much; I don't know if I'll be able to open my eyes in the morning. Will I live through this?

Ultimately, of course, I do. Believe it or not, the next day I feel better! Not *great* but certainly better. If I have one supremely crappy day after every round, I can live with that. I'm looking forward to the next steroid burst.

THE SECOND TREATMENT, THE CONSULT, AND MY SONG

My drive to the cancer center is now familiar. This place that I've hated so determinedly is now a place of hope. It's *my* place, and it's all that can save me. Both cancer diagnoses are no longer a new shock but *part of me*. They are part of my life, though they may be my death. I trust that the people in this place will help.

As a second treatment round bonus, I have no allergic reaction to my mouse infusion! Apparently, the reactions decrease with repeated exposures—the opposite of a bee sting or nut allergy. Who knew?

That steroid euphoria blast felt amazing but not a *real* amazing. This high-energy, no-pain feeling is not a sign of improvement or even evidence of the disease being treated. It is a temporary, phony, steroid-induced amazing. It's gone in eight to ten hours, and meanwhile, I'm just awake. No sleep. I sit up, listen to music, and write while bracing for another day of achy misery and turning once again into a corpse.

When I wake up, I ask my husband to walk the dogs, lie in bed, and assess the lysis misery. It's simply not there. I get up and start my day. I feel great. I'm not achy, nor do I feel tired. My morning progresses without the death snap. I myself take the dogs for their second walk, then am able to take out the trash and recycling without sitting down to rest. This is new. When I walk up the front steps, my legs do not hurt. I don't feel crazy wired from steroids. I just feel *better*.

It may be too soon to be so happy, and it's probably also too soon to have a true disease response. Why do I feel better? Why am I not having the same megadeath cell lysis treatment reaction? I work as usual and continue to feel great.

I realized during this expedition that my cancer needs a soundtrack. Songs pop up in my head at different stages and provide a great deal of solace. You don't select your cancer soundtrack; it selects you. The songs speak and sing to me, and I listen to them on the way to and from my appointments.

I need a triumphant song—a victory song I can blast while fist-pumping, drumming on the steering wheel, and driving. A song that can explode from my phone when I walk out of the cancer center after receiving definitive good news. I need a soundtrack to positive evidence of my cancers succumbing to treatment, for the day I am confirmed to have responded.

> I realized during this expedition that my cancer needs a soundtrack ... you don't select your cancer soundtrack; it selects you.

The song came into my brain without forewarning— "Subdivisions," by Rush. I hadn't heard it in years. Rush—you love them or hate them, and I love them. I love that they're a raw three-piece band with intricate and complex melodies, brisk, crisp drums, soaring vocals, *and* excellent lyrics written by the drummer, of all people. I saw Rush in concert in the midseventies when I was in high school at the Paramount Theater in Austin, Texas. Small venue, magnificent show. Now they're back in my brain.

I love the opening chords. They are freeing. They feel like overcoming obstacles. Not all Rush fans celebrate their synthesizer phase, but "Subdivisions" is now officially the soundtrack for my battle with cancer. Technically, it's a lament to adolescent angst in the suburbs, but that's not what it is for me.

The phrase "mass-production zone" bolted into my head. The line clearly represents the mass IgM production inside me and which is making me sick. The "fringes of the city," the "geometric order," and the "insulated border" perfectly describe the drive I take every time I travel from the foothills to the city, from Conifer to Aurora, from my home to the cancer center.

I meet a new specialist; we'll call him Dr. Second Cancer. He's been billed as exceptional on the topic of Myelo. He tells me that he knows all about my case and has reviewed it carefully and that what I have is not common. He has never seen it, not these two together.

Okay, buddy, pal of mine. You are billed as *the* dude, the beat-all specialist, and you've never seen my condition? As far as he knows, there are no reported cases, ever, of Waldy plus Myelo in the same patient at the same time.

Fortunately for him, I'm feeling great today. He confirms that I do indeed have MDS. He pulls up the final bone marrow pathology report on his computer screen, and there, in bold letters, it is "positive for myelodysplasia." One bone marrow, two cancers. I am a medical phenomenon.

Dr. Second Cancer tells me that he's very comfortable managing this portion of my marrow disease, Myelo, and my primary oncologist, old Dr. Know-It-All, will remain my primary while managing Waldy.

Please, more information. Is the myelodysplasia harming me now? Do I need additional treatment? Will I become transfusion dependent?

He tells me that my anemia is not severe enough for transfusions and that they will not let things get to that point. My hemoglobin is about eight, and they transfuse if it gets under seven. All the while they'll follow this as closely as possible. Then at some point in my life, I will likely develop leukemia. They will find it early and treat me.

I ask, "So this MDS cannot kill me?"

He replies, "I didn't say that. It *can* kill you, but we will not let it."

In his opinion these two cancers are not related. They are incidentally coexisting. I hope they're happy together.

"Do I need more medication added to my regimen right now?"

"There are two effective medications available, but you do not need them now. There will be more on the horizon. If they fail to work, myelodysplasia is curable with a bone marrow transplant."

Ah, the word I had waited to hear for so long—*curable*. Myelo, cancer number two, is curable! Heck, if I get a bone marrow transplant, that may even wipe out Waldy for good!

Let's be clear. I do not *want* to need a bone marrow transplant, but it may be my cure. Right now we can wait and stay the course. We don't need to add more medications. They will not let it kill me, get more aggressive, or even advance. Together we'll stare this thing down.

He asks if I have possible donors. Oh yes, I have *two* sisters lined up to give me their marrow, ready to be tissue-typed. He says it's better to know sooner rather than later if I indeed have a good sibling match because if I don't, I'll need to avail myself of the donor registry.

Everything he's said since confirming my two cancers has been pure music to my ears.

"Do you have any further questions?"

Yes, I have one.

"You're going to make sure I survive?"

"Yes."

For the first time since I received my diagnosis, I feel I'm going to live.

Okay, just *one* more question. I'd received the exact same medications for the first round as the second. Two days after the first round,

I went through the *bonk*, the day of unbearable misery. I should be feeling like crap today, but instead, I feel great. "Why isn't the second round affecting me the same way?"

Did he ever have an answer to that one. He told me the reason I felt so horrible after the first round was due to the billions of cancer cells releasing their toxic cancer *schmetz*—my word—as they died inside of me. The lymphoma mass in my marrow was making me extra sick as a parting gift as it died and departed. My body was then assaulted by dead cancer cell debris, then had to clear out the profusion of dead cells and their toxic contents. Oof. Waldy was dying a billion deaths inside me.

Dr. Second Cancer went on to say that up to 90 percent or more of my cancer cells were killed by that first round and that remaining future cycles are merely "mopping up" to get rid of as many of the remaining 10 percent as possible. What I'd endured was effective treatment. It was my cancer being killed.

Then he mentioned that my hemoglobin had gone up 1.3 points since the first round, which is excellent.

"We are not going to give you more medications and cannot promise you an improved hemoglobin beyond what you're already achieving. There's no need to cause you additional fatigue from additional medications. Your lymphoma doctor called this right from the start. I think you're feeling better because of the reduced tumor burden, and you're getting better."

"Can you please repeat that?"

"I think you are getting better."

I added, as a parting shot, that I would always be interested in clinical trials. At this suggestion, his face turned more serious.

"You will never be accepted into a clinical trial. With two malignant processes never before seen together, there are too many confounding factors. It would be impossible to assess response or symptoms related to one or the other."

I'd suspected this. I have my own personal beliefs about my two cancers, and it's conjecture, not science: I think they're related, but we haven't figured out the connection. I also believe that there is someone else out there with these two together, but we simply haven't found them.

The MDS was not reported on my initial bone marrow report; it was only uncovered after brilliant old Dr. Know-It-All dug deeper. Most doctors, understandably, stop at one cancer, and mine did not.

It isn't yet time to play "Subdivisions," but I'm in decent field position.

I practically sprint down the hall, then take the stairs to the lobby. I call my husband and overwhelm him with information. I am convinced I am going to live. I am the happiest two-cancer-having person on the planet.

THE IGM SURGE

I'm getting severe muscle aches in my legs, mainly in the quadriceps, and as I try to move the laundry from the washer to the dryer, I become so short of breath that I have to sit down on the floor. Then come immediate flashbacks: doing the laundry seems to be triggering my original symptoms.

The leg muscle pain worsens until it's there all the time: at rest, lying down, walking, even for only short distances. I can no longer walk up the front steps without pain. I was leaning over and kneeling in front of the dryer in the same way I'd been leaning over and kneeling on the side of the mountain bike trail.

Six months before my diagnosis, I went for a mountain bike ride with my husband at Staunton State Park, one of our favorites. There, the Borderline Trail has a flowing, easy approach, then a brief transition to steep uphill switchbacks. I had trained myself to ride up all the switchbacks without getting off or putting a foot down, but on that day, I could not do the small ups and downs on the approach. I had ridden less than two miles on easy terrain, and on top of the pain in my legs, I was profoundly short of breath.

Again, I'd written it off, refused to pay attention, then downplayed it. There was clearly something wrong, but it had to happen a few times before it got my attention. Now sitting on the floor in front of my dryer, it officially has my attention. What the heck is going on? I'm supposed to be getting better!

41

Analyzing my disease, trying to match macro symptoms with microbiologic causes, is consuming me. I try to picture what's happening microscopically, deep inside the marrow and my bloodstream, and try to correlate the state of the civilization in my marrow with what I'm feeling. This, to me, is a helpful, brain-occupying coping mechanism.

I go to pick up my seventeen-year-old from skiing. He says he had a great powder day, then says he needs to tell me something. This usually means that he needs new gear or that he lost or broke something on the mountain.

On this occasion he tells me one of the best things I have ever heard in my life, something that made cancer worth it: he says that he misses skiing with me and that he feels bad that I've not been able to go. He wants me to ski with him.

> I want him to remember the great powder days, not the winter his mom had cancer. I will ski with him again.

I tell him that I will not be able to ski this season because I'll be receiving weekly treatments through the beginning of April. I do not want him to feel guilty about skiing without me.

I remind him that we've skied together since he was two. He remembers. I remember. I want him to have fun. I want him to remember the great powder days, not the winter his mom had cancer. I will ski with him again.

THE LAB RESULTS

Here comes the flood
Anything to thin the blood
These corrosives do their magic slowly

—R.E.M., "E-BOW THE LETTER"

My blood draw today gives me my new IgM level, the first since my diagnosis. It's now over three thousand, significantly higher than two thousand, my number when this all started. IgM for a normal, healthy people is in the two hundred to three hundred range. I am baffled.

Just as I need expert advice, in walks the oncology nurse practitioner. These people know so much. She asks about my symptoms, and I tell her about the leg aches and shortness of breath. She says that these are caused by the hyperviscosity from elevated IgM. My blood is too thick and not flowing well into my muscles and lungs. Okay, that makes sense. It's what I've been told from the beginning about IgM. But *why* is the IgM higher? It's my main cancer marker. Shouldn't it go lower as I get treated?

I may have exhibited a bit of rage. She tells me, like so many others before her, that the IgM is a *very large* protein molecule, and as such, it does not immediately filter out of the bone marrow. Last week, when all those cells exploded and died, IgM was released, and it made sludge inside of my marrow.

The sludge takes a long time to exit the bone marrow and enter the bloodstream. When it does seep out of the marrow, it takes another interminable while to be filtered through the kidneys and then finally flushed out of the body. Right now, as it flows out of the marrow and into the bloodstream, it's causing an IgM surge, though I'd call it more of a tsunami, all of which makes me feel sicker.

I'll just have to wait for it to come down. Once it does, maybe I'll no longer have leg pain or shortness of breath. And maybe thereafter I won't have leg pain with light physical exertion. And then maybe, eventually, I can have my life back. Then I can ride my mountain bike to the top of the Borderline Trail without getting off on the switchbacks. *That's* my target IgM level.

Dr. Know-It-All reviews my labs and my newly elevated IgM and tells me that not enough time has elapsed to see real change. He does not want the absence of clear good news to disappoint or upset me, so he suggests not checking my lab values for a while. I've been placed in lab result time-out. Disappointed? Upset? I bite my tongue.

My next bossy oncology nurse is unflappable and fearless. I really want my labs to be drawn. It has been a few weeks, and she just says no. I do not argue. She has needles, equipment, toxic chemicals, and access to a massive database; no one would find my body.

I'm clinging to my results to an extent that they think is bad for my mental health. I guess I'll get the lab draws when I have a contractual agreement with the staff to not have an adult tantrum. Punitive, if you ask me. At least my general well-being has improved over several weeks. I am less tired, weak, sore, and achy.

But there have been a few wake-up calls. While walking the dogs, my typically plodding Newfoundland sprinted up the hill to the neighbor's house. Out of reflex, I tried to run after him and immediately discovered that I could not—too sore, weak, and short of breath.

I'd been thinking about taking longer walks at open space parks and going to the gym to rebuild strength, but clearly I'm not ready.

To other patients, be aware: steroids do create emotional calamities. Cliff dives follow the elevations. I have rough, droopy days where I'm shaky and weepy, even though I otherwise feel quite a bit better. I find it useful to remind myself that these emotions are not me; it's the steroids. I tell myself, "You wept when the yolk broke in the fried egg this morning, but you moved on. It's just the steroids making you a bit nuts. *You're* not nuts. There's a difference." Please do not solicit my husband's opinion on this topic.

Next, I developed a new complication, and was it *ever* a joy; it was as if a sewer rat crawled into my gastrointestinal tract—huge with a thick tail, huge whiskers, and gross teeth. Whatever it was that took up a home in my abdomen, it looked like a pregnancy developing in time-lapse. If I had a bite of food, it did not move; it sat there and decayed while the rat feasted on it. Eventually, he moved on. I suspect the chemo vaporized him. In the process, there were moments of volcanic, gaseous, gnarly eruptions. My husband saluted me in the morning. "There is no way there could possibly be any more gas in your body."

Several rounds in, my fifteen-year-old son asked if he could come with me to my treatment. He heard me telling a friend that I liked having someone there to talk to. I had not asked my kids to join me and had no plans to make them sit there with me in the cancer center. When he asked if he could come, I was beyond touched. When I told him it's going to be boring, he said he was interested in the process and wants to see the place where I spend so much time and to just keep me company.

When we get there, he watches everything and, after every round of nurse-induced torture, never fails to ask, "Hey, Mom, did that hurt?"

After receiving a hall pass from lab time-out, my results are dismal. My hemoglobin is making no further progress, and my IgM is still high. I ask the oncology nurse if he thinks my initial hemo-globin improvement was a temporary surge and whether I was too optimistic. His answer is yes. When I ask him what to expect, he tells me to be patient. My son helpfully interjects that I am not patient. Thanks, sweetie.

Alone, I would not have been very brave after receiving these lab values but was able to be brave for my son. I'm so glad he was there. He's tough. He hiked Angels Landing in Zion National Park with his arm in a cast. You have to use chains to hang on for a few choice stretches near the top there to prevent from falling, so he had one hand on the chain and one in the cast. Unsafe parenting? Perhaps. But he was very clear that he was *not* about to miss that hike.

My legs still hurt, and I'm still dizzy, weak, and tired, and my heart is racing. I kneel on the floor while doing the dishes and laundry, rest between tasks, and kneel outside while walking the dogs. My husband thinks I am getting better. He tells me that, though I may not notice it, I'm sleeping less in the day than I used to and look less pained and weak.

I have Dr. Know-It-All's phone number. I'm tempted to call and say, "Hi! Good morning! How's it going? Are you up? Great! Me too. Thanks to all the medication you keep ordering your sadistic nurses to pump into me, I am up, up, up. Dude, when are you going to publish a case report about me so we can find the one other poor schmuck who also has these two bone marrow cancers? I know they're out there. I can't possibly be the only one. Good night, I mean, morning."

Then more good news: tests confirm that my situation is due to two random, nonhereditary genetic mutations. One genetic mutation for each cancer. Good news for my sisters and children: they have not, will not, and cannot inherit this. How common is Myelo? Four in one hundred thousand in the United States. Ah, these special friends in my bone marrow. My squatters. They're behind on their rent. My expert, non-oncologist opinion: if you, too, have Waldy going on, I'd recommend nudging your oncologist to have a second look at your marrow.

Hesitant as I am to believe it, I feel like I'm improving over a bit more time. I'm always nervous as to whether it will last. Meanwhile, I'm not sleeping as much. I can work, go to the store, *and* cook dinner before I need to lie down. I'm not craving my bed.

As I clear the snow and ice off the car, I feel only slight shortness of breath, like a moderate workout. The car in question is a VW Golf, so there's not too much acreage to clear off, but it was an accomplishment of gargantuan proportions for me. Then later I have to chase the cat across the front lawn, which *did* bring me back to my knees, gasping for breath. At least clearing that snow off the car represents progress. I wonder if other people spend as much time as I do chasing wayward pets.

> Hesitant as I am to believe it, I feel like I'm improving over a bit more time.

BONKERS

I just dropped off my middle and youngest sons with two of their friends at Arapahoe Basin to ski and had to look up at Pallavicini in all its glory. I thought back to my patient, that little boy, skiing it *forty-three* times. Meanwhile, I'm hanging out in the bagel shop, which is kind of sad. I *will* ski A-Basin again.

I love it that my kids are so comfortable in the outdoors. Single- and negative-digit temperatures don't faze them. They have been skiing since they were two. Now it's second nature to them. They have grown up like this: get up early, get your gear together, and face the elements.

As treatments continue, a new era of psychological side effects dawns. The warnings had come from several reliable sources. My doctor recommended an antianxiety sedative and sleep aid from day one of my steroid treatments, and my midlevel providers had all concurred.

I declined, then began staying up much of the night and falling asleep between two thirty and five thirty. Then I progressed to not sleeping at all. Do these darn steroids accumulate? Is there not enough time between doses for them to metabolize before the next assault? Like the chemo, they seem to have a cumulative effect. But while I feel like I've adjusted to the chemo to some extent, it seems like I'm doing the opposite with the steroids.

I look normal, but my mind is going at three thousand miles per hour. I'm writing, working on my business, and taking patient calls.

I try to watch as many sports events as I can on my computer—the NFL playoffs, BMX Vegas Nationals, the early rounds of the Australian Open. I have various electronic devices performing multiple functions. As I do all of these things, I try to convince myself that it's normal.

The next day I realize that I've slept five hours in the past seventy-two. I'm plagued by negative thoughts: *I should stop treatment. I am not fun or active. I'm no good for my family. Cancer has taken my health, my sports, my family.* My thoughts seem to form in a pressure cooker. The cancer treatment is taking over my brain. The inside of my skull feels like it's full of hamsters running on their wheels in every direction.

Later that night I quietly leave my house when everyone is asleep, in the dark, on foot, because I'm not safe to drive. I walk out to the highway thinking I can make it to town to find a hotel in which to sleep until I figure this all out. I don't want to bother my family. I am a burden. Why would they want to deal with me? The nearest hotel is in twenty-five miles or so. Sure, I can make that.

I climb over the highway median cables. I am walking, exhausted, kneeling periodically in the snow beside the highway. At least one concerned motorist saw this spectacle unfolding and helpfully called in a report to the sheriff's hotline. "Um, a woman is walking alone in the dark along the highway, occasionally sitting in the snow on the side of the road. You might want to send someone out."

Soon, the sheriff's deputy pulls up behind me, pats me down, performs a sobriety test, and asks what I am doing. I respond, crying, that I am overtired and have been sick. She so very kindly makes sure that I am okay, then takes me home. I'd not gotten very far, maybe two miles. I'm exhausted. Nuts. Crackers. My mind is gone.

In the morning I wake up and fake normal, make breakfast, go to work, focus on my patients, and push the insanity to the periphery.

Then I call the clinic. I tell them that I am thinking about stopping treatment because the steroids are making me crazy, that I am no good for my family, and that I am losing my mind.

All of those coping skills about which I have been so pompous and proud have broken down. I am mentally unwell. I need help. I am scared I have lost my mind. I continue to sob uncontrollably to the poor intake nurse on the phone, but this is her job, and she is good at her job. She says this steroid reaction is common, predictable, and caused by my medications. She says we must start a strong sedative to calm my brain. We will use the medication appropriately and monitor consistently. We do not want to stop my steroid treatment; it's an integral part of nuking my lymphoma.

I concede defeat and take the sedating medications. I get in bed, take the meds, and sleep for twelve hours. I'm a little groggy the next day but calm. My thoughts no longer race, I'm not paranoid, and I'm no longer convinced my family wants to get rid of me. Fortunately, I'm also not wandering the highway in the dark and snow. Progress!

> Take care of your mental health as you do your physical health.

I call the clinic, give them the report, and make sure I can have another treatment. I can. They are accustomed to dealing with nutjobs like me. I tell the wonderful intake nurse how much better I feel. I feel calm and focused. She says, "Perfect, that's what we do! We call it a factory reset."

Ah, much like cleaning out my marrow and refilling it with the good juice, they wiped my mind clean with steroids and sleep deprivation until not one lucid thought remained. Next, they sedated me to the level of a dead rock star at the bottom of a swimming pool and pushed reboot, and now I'm good to go.

I will go through the same process in advance of my next round to prevent another seventy-two hours of Cirque du Soleil in my brain. There is a place for these medications, and that place is called "temporary insanity." The lesson here: Take care of your mental health as you do your physical health.

I take my crazy-be-gone medication before bed and sleep wonderfully. My prior approach—pushing through the night wide awake— was not tenable long term. Use psych medicines properly, as they may be necessary. If one's not a good fit, your providers will try another. Follow mental symptoms as closely as physical ones.

Be honest, not proud. Keep yourself safe from yourself. You cannot always manage your own case. Medical science has options for mental health treatment. It was pompous and unrealistic of me to make a *goal* out of avoiding mental health medication. Care for and treat it the same as you care for your cancer.

My next treatment nurse practitioner is a to-the-point, no-messing-around professional. Again, I'm allowed to get labs. My hemoglobin is still low, and she tells me that I must stop obsessing over my hemoglobin. I don't see this as an accurate depiction of my refined thought processes, but she can have it her way.

She says the ups and downs of my hemoglobin are meaningless blips. The ups don't mean that I'm better, and the downs don't mean that I'm worse. I should not even *look* at the numbers for now.

I know the word that's about to come out of her vicious mouth: patient. I need to be *patient*. She tells me that we're not even close yet. Again, "Stop looking at your hemoglobin." I promise that I will try.

Then this particularly sinister nurse practitioner asks, "Are you aware that you have a really big molecule?"

THE LAB-INDUCED CONFUSION

If I wait for just a second more
I know, I'll forget what I came here for

—YAZOO, "NOBODY'S DIARY"

Today is a sad day in the Blood Disorders Infusion Center. There is a new patient whom I have not seen here before, a young woman who appears to be in her thirties. It's always sad to see someone here so young. I still think of *myself* as so young, yet she appears twenty years younger.

Then there's another gentleman, maybe in his forties, that I've seen here several times. He looks much worse today. He has that telltale pale, bronze-green-orange facial color, and he looks tired. I would love to be able to tell him that I hope he gets better and that I'm sorry he's so sick.

Still, not one of us cancer patients ever break the social barrier. We *see* each other but do not make eye contact.

My IgM comes back at 2,960. Almost no progress at all and still higher than at the time of my diagnosis. Does this mean I'm not responding? This is all Waldy's fault; he makes the IgM, not Myelo. He was *supposed* to have been 90 percent demolished. If treatment is working, my IgM should be down. I fear that I'm in the 30 percent nonresponder group and do not know the next step if that is the case. Push ahead, I guess, but for what? Why can't I get rid of my big stupid molecule?

I arrive at home droopy and gloomy. Our Newfoundland, Picasso, greets me. He's old for a large breed but healthy, loves his walks, and does not act sick, but he's getting a little nutty. He barks early in the morning at five o'clock to let us know he's ready to get his day started. I have a dear friend who's a vet, and she performs in-home, compassionate pet euthanasia. As I enter the house looking down in the dumps, bitching about my elevated IgM, my husband asks me if I think my vet friend would give us a two-for-one deal on me and Picasso. This explains why we have been married for twenty-five years.

In the end that sewer rat has not returned, my insanity has been replaced with logical thought, and my sleep cycle has normalized. All of these are successful interventions, yet my IgM, *the* most important barometer of my response to treatment, is not only barely budging but also getting worse. Every Waldy help site informs me that the IgM should go down within three or so months, and I've already been at it for longer than that.

Why am I managing all of these side effects if my cancer is not being treated? I await the response from my contact nurse, who will be discussing this with Dr. Know-It-All. I still have his cell phone number, but I am still not yet ready to abuse the privilege. When they finally acknowledge that I'm toast, maybe I'll finally call him up.

Then later the bone marrow transplant coordinator calls with spectacular news: if I need a bone marrow stem cell transplant, both of my sisters are 100 percent matches. Generally, a full biological sibling will have a 25 percent chance of being a full match, so to have 200 percent matches is fortunate to say the least. I hope I don't need their marrow, but meanwhile, they're ready to donate if and when I do. The terms "bone marrow transplant" and "stem cell transplant" are used interchangeably. Bone marrow transplant is the original, older term. Stem cell transplant is the more modern and accurate term. More on this later.

Dr. Know-It-All will call tomorrow for a thirty-minute phone conference. Market research has demonstrated that thirty minutes is the appropriate amount of time to professionally and compassionately tell a patient their treatment is failing and that they are going to croak. I wonder what he'll have to say about my IgM.

THE INFORMATION

At every occasion, I'll be ready for the funeral.
—BAND OF HORSES, "THE FUNERAL"

Dr. Yapper Know-It-All calls at noon on the dot, and I barely get a word in edgewise. The guy talks more than I do. He says that he *does* wish that my IgM was lower at this point, and it hits me like a cannonball in the gut. He admits that there is not much data on this topic because Waldy is so rare. IgM simply may take longer to clear in some patients, and it does not necessarily mean they're not responding. A quarter or so of patients may see their IgM surge for up to four months before it finally decreases. None of this is comforting.

We're going to give it another four weeks to see if the IgM does eventually decrease. He tells me that my immune system is not perfect "in a few different directions." How poetic. Maybe *he* should be writing my book. Do I understand and agree with the plan? Oh sure.

I finish with my own patients throughout the afternoon, then talk to my husband. We have a plan. We are going to stay the course. Then later my husband calls me back. He is worried that he and the boys will not have much time with me and that my leukemia treatment is not working. I reply that I am not getting treated for leukemia, as I do not exactly have that yet. I am being treated for *lymphoma*. He says, "Fine, if you have to get technical."

The poor dear has no idea what illnesses I actually have. He is so focused on me as a person and my survival that he truly *does not know*. This is a precious quality. I think he knows "cancer," "oncologist," and "bone marrow," and that's about the extent of it. I very much doubt he knows Waldenström's or myelodysplasia or which is which.

I tell him how much better I am feeling overall and that I'm looking forward to the day when I no longer have aching legs and shortness of breath. To this he says, "You're short of breath?" This is either a testament to my lack of whining about symptoms or an excellent example of him not listening to me. This is coming from the man who had our kids fill out their own census forms because he couldn't remember their birthdates, so I'll leave this one up to you.

I assure my husband that Dr. Oncotron Know-It-All has plans B through Z ready but that I'm not ready to hear about them because I want plan A to work. I am fully committed to plan A. Plan B is a daily medication that I would have to take in perpetuity.

"I will survive this," I say. My husband is reassured. I remind him what a comfort he has been throughout this and what a comfort it is to know that the boys have him. I know every day that our three sons will be fine. He remains calm.

Then I clear the snow off the truck, crank the heat and Band of Horses's "The Funeral," and cry. I wail, moan, and scream out loud in the truck. "How can I have two cancers? How is this possible? I'm so young. I'm so healthy. I ski extreme terrain. I've climbed all the four-teeners except one. I race BMX! We *must* beat these cancers. We must!"

I sob through the song, then shake, slap, and snap myself back into reality and drive to the store. I cannot fall apart. Cancer or not, we still need groceries for dinner.

THE OSCILLATIONS

You know the way
It throws about
It takes you in
And spits you out
It spits you out
When you desire
To conquer it ...
Oh, cuts you up

—PETER MURPHY, "CUTS YOU UP"

They send my labs to my phone, and I'm not supposed to look, but of course, I can't help myself.

After plodding along at eight and nine for so long, my hemoglobin is eleven! I burst into tears of sheer joy. This is the best it's been in ten months, well before my diagnosis. Before I knew about my IgM, this was my original problem and obsession. I call my husband from my bay immediately, and he's so happy. I can feel the sigh of relief in his voice. My lab values have also become the barometer of *his* happiness.

I go to the bathroom so as not make a scene in the treatment area. I am sobbing a Hallmark movie sob loudly, repeating aloud, "It's an eleven. It's an eleven. My hemoglobin is an eleven." I never thought I would see eleven again. After some time I regain some semblance of composure and return to my bay.

My oncology nurse practitioner today is very happy with my progress. I have no physical complaints, I'm on a good sleep schedule, and my energy is high, though I'm still not able to exert myself much physically. While I'm thrilled with my hemoglobin, I'm still grumpy about my IgM, and we'll have to wait a few weeks for another reading. I ask him what he thinks about it still being elevated at the last check.

"I'm not sure if you're aware, but this is a very big protein molecule."

A family calls my office to say their six-year-old daughter is having difficulty breathing. This, of course, is a bring-in. She walks in with pronounced, heavy hyperventilation. She looks parched and is tired enough to lie down on my exam table rather than sitting. Her interaction and mental status are poor. Most of all, her respiratory pattern is distinctive. The diagnosis is already made. This is diabetic ketoacidosis, a complication of juvenile diabetes—a lifelong illness. She and her parents have no idea.

I do a quick confirmation with a urine dipstick and a finger poke glucose test. I have a bedside confirmation within minutes. After the diagnosis, I information-dump on her parents and arrange ambulance transport to intensive care.

Looking back, their child had been wetting the bed, drinking and voiding way more than baseline, and looking thinner and thinner. They had not put it all together, but why would they? For now putting parental guilt to rest is the most important thing I can do. Months later her parents have encyclopedic diabetes knowledge, love their pediatric endocrinologist, and most importantly their child is fine. I love my job every day, but I particularly love days like these.

Later in the week, I see a teen who has been chronically running away from home and school. He's in a special school that supports his cognitive and mental health challenges. Unfortunately, he's also facing obesity. I asked him what he thought he could do for exercise. He told me he wants to run and wants to start with ten-mile trail runs.

Of course, this is not a realistic plan. Too high of an initial goal will result in failure. I suggest that he work up to this trail run by starting with a walk, then a brisk walk, and then a walk-run.

He lights up and says he knows all about the walk-run because this is what he does when he runs away from school. He and his friends start out at a walk, then break into a run when the school calls the cops. This isn't exactly what I pictured, but it works. His father, sister, and I all break out laughing. He's happy that he made us laugh.

After more treatments and more labs, my email dings with a new test result. My IgM is 1,819—over a thousand point drop since last time. There it is. I look at it over and over to make sure it's real. The big, dumb, fat, stupid protein molecule made by this stupid lymphoma is going down. I'm a responder!

I've been waiting for this since my diagnosis and was no longer sure that I'd ever see it happen. Four-plus months after my first treatment, my IgM is going down. It is not normal or even close to normal, but it's *going down.*

I have been wrong about many things in this illness. I was wrong when I thought for months that hemoglobin was the key lab value. I was wrong when I thought my anemia was the biggest factor in how sick I felt. And I was wrong when I believed that I would not need mental health support or sleep, that I'd sail through treatment without complications and when I assumed I could will my way through the myriad side effects. Wrong, wrong, wrong.

I did manage to stick to my single most important goal, however: this dumb, stupid, uninvited cancer did not have a massive negative impact on my family. This never became "the year that Mom got cancer." Even when I was in bed for hours or days at a time, I was there. My kids went on with their lives as they otherwise would have. My cancer was not the centerpiece topic of family discussions. We talked about it only if they asked or if there was a significant good or bad report. I am proud that I exhibited bravery and that my kids saw it.

In the end I only missed two days of work, both of which were for all-day infusions, never from feeling too sick. I went to work the day after the eleven-hour infusion and death-corpse night. I will always be proud of this.

I was so depressed for the first few days after my diagnosis, but it got better. Fighting through gives way to perseverance, knowledge, savvy information gathering, trust in medical professionals, and realizing that experts are there to help at every step. Remember, the depression does not last. The initial days of intense gloom are finite. The frantic searching for the cure, looking for the website that says you will live? It ends.

> When people ask how I got through, my response is simple: keep going. I got out of bed every morning, put my foot on the floor, and thought, *Go, go, go.*

In its place, a more realistic journey begins. It's been a long haul over the last six months, with so many ups and downs. You can't escape the cliché—there are so many ups and downs, sometimes in the same day or even the same hour. Five months of weekly treatment—my first treatment was on November 27, 2018, and the last was on April 27, 2019. When people ask how I got through, my response is simple: keep going. I got out of bed every morning, put my foot on the floor, and thought, *Go, go, go.*

An elderly gentleman, perhaps in his eighties, is at the infusion center on my last day there. He has that cancer color and is getting a blood transfusion. He's pushing his IV pole, as I am, and his gets stuck on the entranceway to the bathroom. He turns to me and says, "That was the first thing I learned: to lower the IV pole to enter the bathroom." We both laugh. He, too, is just trying to *keep going*. He looks happy. I can see he has more life to live.

Is it too sentimental to say that cancer has been, and will continue to be, a positive thing in my life? Could that possibly be true?

Yes, it can.

In the end it *has* been positive. I have beaten it as much as I can for now. In the process I have felt my own strength. Now that I've lived through it, I hope I can use it to help others.

Throughout this entire process, I never allowed myself to listen to the entirety of "Subdivisions." Only bits and pieces: the geometric order; the far, unlit unknown; the mass-production zone; the lit up like a firefly feeling the living night. Finally, when my treatment course was complete and I had definitively positive news, I allowed myself to listen to the whole song—again and again.

I stand before you—Waldy, Myelo, and me coexisting. My doctors and I will watch them like hawks. They will not rear back up and take over. At this point they cannot aggress. If they so much as try, we will aggress back.

THE CLOSING ARGUMENTS

Saw things so much clearer
Once you were in my rearview mirror
I gathered speed from you fucking with me
Once and for all
I'm far away
Hard to believe
Finally the shades are raised

—PEARL JAM, "REARVIEWMIRROR"

I meet with Dr. Know-It-All for a posttreatment recheck. He thinks that I'm doing great, which translates to *not dead*. He thinks it will be good for me to exercise lightly, for brief periods, in pursuit of reasonable goals. Check.

I ask him if he thinks my IgM will get below one thousand, as I'm still stagnating in the mid-one-thousand range. He says he does not know. I ask if he thinks my hemoglobin will ever recover. He says he does not know. I then want to ask if he ever went to oncology school, but I appreciate the uncertainties and the honesty.

I go to Santa Fe with my middle son and one of his friends for an enduro bike race, and there, I ride a bike for the first time since 2018. Thirty minutes of easy terrain. This is huge. I feel sadness pondering how the year's events unfolded, and as I ride, it's replaced by optimism for the future. I rode my bike, and that is enough.

It doesn't get much worse than the day of that phone call in Gunnison. Or the day of that eleven-hour, allergy-laden infusion. Or learning that I had a second cancer. But I got better. I will live with cancer. I will maybe even find another human out there with my two bone marrow malignancies. C'mon, Waldy. C'mon, Myelo. Let's go.

PART II
STRAIGHT INTO HELL

THREE MONTHS LATER—
THE WALKOUT

Crying won't help you, praying won't do you no good

—LED ZEPPELIN, "WHEN THE LEVEE BREAKS"

"**I** have patients much sicker than you," says Dr. Gatekeeper, leaning back in his chair while fondling his comb-over.

"I'm sure you have," I respond. "You take care of the sickest patients in the hospital, but that is an irrelevant point and does not render my illness less worthy of your care."

"I consider a stem cell transplant to be a salvage procedure. You need to try more treatments and be more critically ill."

"I prefer to not wait until I need to be salvaged. Have you ever treated a patient with my combination of bone marrow cancers?"

"No."

"Have you reviewed the treatment regimen that I've completed?"

"Yes, and it has been only one treatment regimen. It is not enough. You need to take two new medications: one for the Waldenström's lymphoma and one for the myelodysplastic syndrome."

I was in decent shape for three months after completion of treatment. I did not feel horribly sick every day, did not ache all the time, and was not short of breath after low exertion. I could jog, though it was more like a slow plod, for three miles of flat terrain. I could ride my bike for almost an hour, if not too steep, and I could handle the blue runs at the downhill bike park with obvious help from gravitational pull. I could take trips with my family. I could go to bike races—though as a spectator, no longer a competitor. I could walk uphill for a short period, if not at too much of an incline. The leg pain and shortness of breath returned with anything more than minimal exertion, though I figured that would get better with conditioning. I did have to call one of my sons on two occasions to pick me up when I could not ride back home.

All of this was better than lying in bed and feeling cancer-sick and ache-addled. I could live comfortably this way. I could coexist with Waldy and Myelo. We could all three live in some strange kind of harmony, and meanwhile, I would work on my exercise tolerance.

Alas, it wasn't to be. I started to have days where I planned to get out and walk or ride, but when I tried, I could not. I started to feel feverish and sickly, like I was getting influenza. I sobbed in pain at night with aches in my legs and lower back. I was tired. At first I downplayed the symptoms, just as I had done when they first appeared. I thought to myself, *I have a viral illness*, or *I am tired*, or *I am having a bad day*, or simply *I am achy*.

> Diagnostic gymnastics were not required to find the answer. Deep down, I knew it. Reaccepting it was the challenge.

You idiot! It was obviously the cancer. You were not cured, your improvements were not being sustained, and you were deteriorating. You *knew* this. Diagnostic gymnastics were not required to find the answer. Deep down, I knew it. Reaccepting it was the challenge. The precise, evidence-based decisions and my five months of treatments had simply not worked.

I still had two doctors that I loved. Dr. Know-It-All was in charge of Waldy, and Dr. Second Cancer handled Myelo. They listened. They put an incredible amount of thought into each decision. We thoroughly discussed our collective plan. They communicated with each other. We had decided to treat Waldy first, and aggressively, as the lymphoma was most likely responsible for my more severe symptoms.

When my symptoms reappeared, Dr. Know-It-All felt I could try an oral medication for the lymphoma. It has many serious side effects, and I thought it seemed like a better option for someone much older. It also didn't seem like a good option for long-term use. It's not curative, the disease rebounds when you stop taking it, the side effects range from mild to life-altering to fatal. Plus, it doesn't treat Myelo.

Dr. Know-It-All agreed that discussing a transplant was reasonable but thought I should consider the drug to see if I would tolerate and respond to it. I respected his opinion. I asked Dr. Second Cancer if we should consider treating Myelo. Maybe it was a bigger player than we thought. A chromosomal abnormality puts me in a 10 percent subtype of Myelo patients who are treatable.

The word "treatable" is subject to interpretation, but I was ready to try. Dr. Second Cancer said that the medication would likely increase my hemoglobin and therefore treat my anemia but would not be a *cure*. It would probably not help me feel less achy or less sick, has a litany of severe side effects, and does not prevent Myelo from progressing to leukemia.

Well, that makes it essentially useless. My assessment of the drug went from "treatment" to "useless" as if descending a waterslide.

Myelo will become leukemia. That is simply what it does. *When* it does, it kills you. It can happen at any time and aggressively. Dr. Second Cancer did not think that this "treatment" was the way to

69

go. Eliminating the possibility of developing leukemia was, to me, the only type of treatment that made sense. I wanted to work toward a transplant.

To this he said, "You are thinking about this in the right way, and I think that is what you need. It is a *cure*, and it would likely cure the lymphoma as well."

Perfect. Let us proceed.

He then uttered the fateful words. "You will be transferred to a new doctor, and he will take over your care."

That meant no more Dr. Know-It-All and no more Dr. Second Cancer, both of whom had been with me since the start, taking amazing care of me.

This is how I end up face-to-face with Dr. Gatekeeper, their only transplant doctor. I tell him that Dr. Second Cancer does not think medication is a good option and that I agree it won't help much in the long term. I'd already been through a lot of medications. None of my current choices are a cure, *except* for getting a stem cell transplant.

In response Dr. Gatekeeper launches into the risks of transplantation. He tells me I have an 80 percent chance of graft-versus-host disease (GVHD). This is where the new, transplanted stem cells get overexcited, drive out of their lane, and start attacking their host—me—via the skin, liver, mouth, eyes, and gastrointestinal tract. Severe, long-term symptoms are a huge risk.

I ask if the percentage improves with a good match and excellent underlying health. Other than this little problem of having two cancers, I am fine, and I have a 100 percent match from not one but two sisters. I also ask how much of GVHD is severe and lifelong and how much is mild and can be treated.

"The statistics on that are complex."

I tell him that I believe that any patient researching their options should at least be given a shot at understanding pertinent "complex statistics." As patients, we have our doctors, and we have Google.

Then he says, "Most of the patients here that receive a transplant regret that they ever got one and would prefer to have their disease back."

If that were true, I do not believe this splendid gentleman would have a transplant program to be in charge of in the first place. I still don't believe it. I believe he was simply trying to talk me out of it.

"Additionally," he explains, "you will need to find someone to be your caregiver posttransplant. This person needs to agree to care for you, drive you to your appointments, learn your medications, care for your indwelling intravenous line, be prepared to bring you to the hospital at a moment's notice, and monitor you for complications. It can be a taxing job."

At this point I become apoplectic to the point where I cannot verbally respond. I am here with my husband. *Husband.* Sickness and health. We've had twenty-five years of health, and now we're dealing with sickness. I do not even need to ask my husband if he's up to the task. He doesn't have more important plans on his calendar, and I do not need to "find someone" to be my caregiver. I have one. He came preregistered.

Dr. Gatekeeper says that his "offer" is to put me on the two medications previously discussed.

I ask, "Have you ever had a patient on both these medications, each with multiple dangerous side effects, at the same time?"

"No."

"Are you aware of any medical literature or case reports of a patient on both of these medications, long term, at the same time?"

"No."

71

"Then I will agree to try these medications, one at a time, in preparation for a transplant but not in the place of a transplant."

"No. That is not what we are going to do. You must take both medications to attempt to treat both cancers, and you are not approved for transplant. We are not headed in that direction."

"May I review this with my doctors who have known me for a year?"

"I can talk to them for you."

"What do you see as the natural progression of my MDS?"

"You will develop leukemia."

"I'm young. I want my life back," I plead. "I'm willing to accept the risks of a transplant, and I believe that my opinion should carry some weight in this conversation. I do not think that these other options are a good long-term plan. It's a lifelong commitment to two medications not typically taken together, each with high risk of severe side effects, no cure, and no protection from leukemia."

I continued, "Plus, no one can assess how sick I feel except *me*. I feel sick every day, all the time, and have for well over a year. My legs ache. My back aches. I feel tired and flu-like all the time. I'm up most nights writhing with leg pain. I am short of breath, exhausted, and it gets worse with minimal exertion. Right now my general health is excellent. The transplant will be riskier and possibly less effective if we wait until I'm older, sicker, and weaker. It makes no sense to me to wait. I *will* need this transplant at some point. Now is the time."

"And that is precisely why I am not approving you. You look too healthy. You *are* too healthy. You can't only hear what you want to hear."

"Oh really? I've *heard* that I have one rare cancer, a second rare cancer, that I'll go through months of immunotherapy infusions, chemotherapy, and steroids, and then despite everything, I've *heard* that I'm *still* sick. Both of my cancers are still present in my bone marrow biopsy, and it's been six months since I completed treatment. Since I walked through these doors, I've only heard things that I do *not* want to hear. Do I need to wail in pain and writhe on the floor to convince you?"

Then I walk out. I do not trust this guy. Instead of inquiring about how my symptoms are affecting my life, he's discounting them. He cannot make the case that I'm malingering—this very institution, his employer, found *both* cancers. How can it be possible that I have two intensely symptomatic, potentially fatal cancers in my bone marrow yet still need to work so hard to convince this transplant physician that they're making me sick?

This center quickly diagnosed and took excellent care of me. I trust my two doctors and the nurses. I love seeing the check-in staff, who are so kind. But I can no longer have my trusted doctors if I wish to proceed with a transplant, and I do not trust Dr. Gatekeeper to take good care of me.

I am out the door and in tears.

THE NEW CLINIC

The Colorado Blood Cancer Institute is my new home away from home. Like anyone else, I googled it, and now here I am, armed with an agenda.

The doctor appears. My husband is hoping I let the poor guy speak and that I do not throw a tantrum and walk out. He supports me unconditionally, but Dr. Gatekeeper effectively terrified him out of the transplant, and he is now hyperfocused on his fear of GVHD.

This new doctor is familiar with my case. He has reviewed my records, knows my treatments, and takes great interest in my current symptoms. I give him the same speech about how I've been feeling over the past year plus. "I am an impostor in my own life. I am here with the goal of receiving a stem cell transplant. It's my only hope for a cure."

I've come full circle—from wanting a cure to treating and managing and back to wanting a cure. I do not want to hear about endless treatments. We know more now. I have dedicated immense mental energy into attempting to understand my symptoms and relating those symptoms to the molecular, microbiological happenings inside of me. I cannot figure it all out, and it does not matter anymore. I want it all gone. This new doctor needs to think and revisit my records. I predict an insufficient response and plot a forceful rebuttal.

He says we can proceed in the direction of a transplant, but we will do treatments in preparation to reduce the cancers and evaluate my response. He does not want to do the transplant in the fall, before influenza season. It is much safer in the spring or summer. Meanwhile, we'll wage an aggressive campaign to prevent GVHD.

Great. Perfect. Love it. My husband and I exhale in unison. This man is going to help us.

This new doctor, hereafter known as Dr. Good Ideas, suggests that we try another round of the same immunotherapy infusions I have previously received because they helped debulk Waldy. Meanwhile, we will not do the chemo or the steroids, which I am so relieved to hear; they make me feel great, then make me certifiably bonkers. I do not want to play that game again.

> I do not get exactly what I ideally want, to have the transplant approved by insurance and scheduled for the next few weeks, but I have been heard and am now on the path.

Dr. Good Ideas listens and thinks. I do not get exactly what I ideally want, to have the transplant approved by insurance and scheduled for the next few weeks, but I have been heard and am now on the path.

THE SECOND TAKE

Oh, now I feel it coming back again.

—LIVE, "LIGHTNING CRASHES"

I restart weekly mouse gut immunotherapy infusions, and now I tolerate them very well. I do around eight, but who's counting? I don't even check my labs compulsively anymore. Gone is the cycle of feeling like death and coming back to life. My symptoms and my labs do not improve. Waldy has become resistant to immunotherapy. What a jerk. I continue to ask myself, as all cancer patients ask themselves, how many times and how many ways I can express that cancer sucks and I feel like crap.

As he gets to know me and my symptoms, Dr. Good Ideas believes that Myelo has been significant all along. We hoped that once we cleared Waldy out of my bone marrow, there'd be more room to produce normal red blood cells. Nope. Didn't happen. I hung on to my hemoglobin level with every blood draw, seeing every little budge as a positive trend. It was all false hope. Insignificant blips came right back down. Why? Because Myelo was causing my anemia, and we were not treating Myelo.

Dr. Good Ideas is confident that my backache, fatigue, and general sick feeling are from Myelo and that the leg aches and shortness of breath are from Waldy. It's so hard to know which malignancy is causing which symptoms, and I've finally depleted my mental energy in addressing this question. I never found the answer. I've learned so much yet know so little about my diseases. But I do know that I cannot live with the symptoms of these cancers and that they need to go.

My IgM, my primary lymphoma marker, does not budge after the second series of weekly immunotherapy infusions—no surge, no decrease, nothing. My symptoms are the same, and I am still sick. Now I'm done with immunotherapy infusions for good.

Dr. Good Ideas suggests trying an oral medication for Myelo to see if it helps my anemia. I've already discussed this same medicine with Dr. Second Cancer and Dr. Gatekeeper. Now I feel I have no choice but to take it. If I'm to proceed with the transplant, I have to try everything that can reasonably offer relief. Dr. Good Ideas agrees that this should be the *only* medication I take so we can assess side effects and responses without confusion.

> I do know that I cannot live with the symptoms of these cancers and that they need to go.

Now I have an in-depth interview with the specialty pharmacist to consent to the many and serious risks of this medication. Most of the side effects overlap with my list of cancer symptoms. It's like a two-for-one bonus special! There's no way I'll agree to taking it long term. In any case the medication arrives at my home in a yellow-and-black hazmat bag. I open it and swallow one of the suckers right down.

Over the next few months, the hazmat medication increases my hemoglobin to a normal state after two years of anemia. Precisely as Dr. Second Cancer had predicted, I feel the same. The aches and sick feeling do not abate. Then my platelets and white cells precipitously drop to a dangerous level, and the hazmat medication is stopped. I am glad it is my only medication and that we definitively know it's the culprit.

The life span of a red blood cell is 120 days, so now I can proceed with my transplant without anemia. This is a very good thing. Ultimately, I'm glad that I took it, that it was brief, and that it's over.

LET'S TRY MORE STUPID MEDICATION

There's a battle ahead
Many battles are lost ...
Hey now, hey now
Don't dream it's over

—CROWDED HOUSE, "DON'T DREAM IT'S OVER"

As we're getting closer to the final countdown, Dr. Good Ideas asks if I'll try the other lymphoma medication I've been avoiding. The side effects include bleeding, infections, low white blood cells, abnormal heart rhythm, fatigue, muscle pain, and bone pain. Oh sure. Why the heck not? Again, my treatment is likely to cause the same symptoms as my illness.

Then COVID-19 hits. Dr. Good Ideas is nervous. "If I'm going to treat you, you cannot go to work. You *cannot* risk getting COVID. It would be devastating for you."

I've happily and proudly worked through this entire illness, and now I must stop. By March 2020, I'm home on total lockdown but perform some telemedicine appointments for my patients when appropriate. I have a wonderful nurse practitioner and two indispensable medical assistants. I am forever grateful to them. The office never closes. COVID-19, cancer, whatever—we keep chugging along.

My new lymphoma medication is also shipped from a specialty pharmacy, but it does not arrive in a hazmat bag. It brings my IgM down into the seven hundred range, my lowest level yet. Minimizing Waldy pretransplant is extremely reassuring, but unfortunately, I do not feel better.

For the first year or so, I believed with every synapse in my brain that if I could get my hemoglobin and IgM relatively normal, I would feel great. No medical professional ever told me this; I concocted it in my own mind. Now my lab result fantasy has come true, but I'm still sick. My hemoglobin is normal, and my IgM is below one thousand, but I feel no better.

From here, I have one of many epiphanies to come. I am not supposed to be harboring two cancers in my bone marrow. They are not compatible with life, or feeling good, or maintaining any semblance of daily normalcy. After all that I've learned, for all that I've read, for every lab I've obsessed over, and for all that I've been taught, it's so simple: living with these cancers in the bone marrow is not a functional predicament.

Then my white count drops again to a dangerous level. Is it the medication? The illnesses? Who knows? In any case Dr. Good Ideas says I can stop taking this latest medication. We have beaten Waldy and Myelo down as far as we safely can. I've jumped through every hoop, and now I get my transplant.

THE PRETRANSPLANT
HOME PREP

You leave in the morning with everything
you own in a little black case
Alone on a platform, the wind and the
rain on a sad and lonely face
—BRONSKI BEAT, "SMALLTOWN BOY"

Now there's a crapload of stuff to do: informational video, note-taking, and in-person sessions. I learn that I'll need to change my housecleaning plan. The required-viewing educational transplant process videos provided by the clinic to the patients make a huge point about this. Preventing infectious complications at home post-transplant is a huge deal.

I'm not a great housekeeper. Groceries, cooking, and laundry are my strengths. Dusting, mopping, scrubbing the bathroom? Not so much. I certainly do these things; I do not love them. My husband and my two sons living at home claim that they'll divide up the essential chores; we'll see how this goes. We ultimately hire a weekly house cleaner and schedule a deep clean for when I return. I also hire a service to perform doggie yard cleaning. My husband and sons might *agree* to perform this chore, but I am skeptical that it will happen. We need professionals. I assign duties for the litter box, laundry, dishes, trash, recycling, and mail pickup. Hopefully, they can handle it.

I organize and consolidate my belongings, weed out clothing, and arrange my sports gear. I have so much gear, and I want it to be easy to donate my stuff if I croak. Morbid but reasonable. My kids see the dentist and the eye doctor, then get physicals and any due vaccines. The dogs go to the vet. The bills get paid. I get the house management as current as possible before my departure. All of these are psychologically vital steps. Get the household dialed in before being gone for a month and possibly forever.

I purchase loose sweatpants and loose tops for the hospital, in disastrous color choices. These will prove to be my smartest purchases. I cannot stress this enough: loose sweatpants and loose tops. Nothing constricting *anywhere*. Count on going from being too warm and sweaty to freezing and shivering in rapid succession. Bring layers in a ten-day supply. There's a laundry.

No one wants to be in a hospital gown; it gives one the aura of "chronic invalid." I never once put one on. I also bring comfy, fluffy, fuzzy slippers and get more compliments on them than I could ever imagine. What girl doesn't love having her footwear admired?

I load up my laptop, tablet, and phone and leave the electric toothbrush and floss at home; they're way too rough on the mouth. Get soft, manual toothbrushes. There will be times when even these are too rough, and you go to a soft cloth.

Of course, I bring a hairbrush. Who am I kidding? My hair will eventually fall out in clumps. At a certain point, so much will have fallen out—onto my pillow, into my food, and into the trash can while puking—that I shriek in horror upon seeing my image in the mirror, then ask to have my head shaved. This is preferable, by far. At first I avoid the mirror, then adjust and do not even care. The point is, do not bring a hairbrush.

Saying goodbye is rough. I want to say goodbye to *everyone* but don't want to be too morose. They drill the 15–20 percent mortality rate into your head to the extent that it's always there, lurking. All kinds of things can go wrong. I give my sons my best mom advice: "Don't do stupid crap." I'm confident that my sage counsel was promptly forgotten. I tell them that I have had an amazing, wonderful life, that there is nothing that I want to do that I have not done, and that I want them to be happy.

No visitors are allowed in the bone marrow transplant unit during COVID-19 at any time. I'm sad about this at first, as is my husband. Then the sadness is replaced with relief that no one will witness what I'm about to endure.

An extensive pretransplant medical evaluation is required: comprehensive blood screening for every organ system and function, infection rule-outs, pulmonary function tests, cardiac echo and EKG, chest X-ray, sinus X-ray, dental evaluation and cleaning, psychological and cognitive assessments. I guess I pass!

Under anesthesia, I get a central line with three access ports; it's tunneled under the skin, over the collarbone, and then into the internal jugular vein. The physician's assistant who does this asks if I want to see the line. No, no, and no. I'm already trying to keep the image of the thing popping into

> I tell them that I have had an amazing, wonderful life, that there is nothing that I want to do that I have not done, and that I want them to be happy.

my internal jugular vein out of my mind and have zero interest in seeing it. Please put me out and put the dang thing in. My husband

and I learn how to clean and flush it. I am now officially a full-on transplant patient.

Dr. Good Ideas gives me my final checkup and obtains my consent before sending me to purgatory. It feels more like a business transaction and in no way accurately represents how much this will suck. He's a physician of careful decisions and few words. He tells me, "You look so healthy. There are many transplant doctors who would not agree to perform this transplant."

Oh, I'm certainly aware.

"I understand the risks. I know I can get GVHD despite a perfect match and preventive measures. I know I can develop sepsis and the other potentially fatal complications. I know the transplant may not work. I know I can die. I know all these things. I know what I'm doing. I will never second-guess this decision, and I will never regret it. Never. This is my chance. This is my cure."

We wait until COVID-19 is more under control and ensure the hospital has a handle on precautions. My husband comes with me to admissions but cannot come up to my unit. This is a sad moment.

To the family of a patient, know that you are dropping your loved one off at the gates of hell.

THE HOSPITAL ROOM

As streetlamps pour orange colored
shapes, through your windows
A broken soul stares from a pair of watering eyes
Uncertain emotions force an uncertain smile
—THE THE, "UNCERTAIN SMILE"

The aide carries my belongings, and I follow her down the hall toward the isolated bone marrow transplant unit. My room has an east-facing view of the roof, which reflects an orange tint from the light outside, especially at sunrise. That pretty little flicker of light was a comforting sight in the morning from my hospital bed. When I saw it, I knew I had survived the night and was still alive.

I am relieved to finally be here and to get the party started. I am more excited than scared, but I'm still scared and a little weepy. I will rarely leave this room for the next month, and I know it will be a room of pain.

I have a day before my chemo starts, and am full of goals. I'll be doing in-bed exercises and mile-long walks in the hallways. I plan to keep this up through the entire stay, no matter what. So naive. You'd think by now I would've learned.

A parade of people come to see me: occupational therapy, physical therapy, oncology dietitian, in-house attending physician, physician's assistant, nurse practitioner, nurse, aide, psychologist. I love the visitors and take the opportunity to draw whatever wisdom, experience, and advice I can out of them.

I have a stable of in-house physicians who see me throughout my monthlong stay, and one member of the group checks in on me daily. They each have their own style. I see this as an excellent opportunity to gather more insight into my rare diagnoses and my course thus far.

The first oncologist I see is the only female physician on staff. She reviews my case and asks a question I had never heard. "You received your diagnosis almost two years ago. What took so long for you to get to a transplant?"

My eyebrows shoot up, and my jaw is on the floor.

"I had a hard time getting a transplant physician to agree to the transplant. I had several rounds of treatments first, and then there was a time that I thought I could live with the cancers. When I felt a bit better after my first round of treatment, I thought I could go on living with the cancers and that we could all coexist."

> It has been a long fight to get here. I am ready to be fixed. I am ready to be reborn.

"Carol, that would never have been possible. You would've always been too sick. No human is meant to live with these two malignancies. That was *never* a viable option. This transplant is the only way for you to go."

My relief in hearing her opinion feels like fresh air, a validation I was no longer even seeking. I want to jump up and hug her, but COVID-19 precautions preclude it.

It has been a long fight to get here. I am ready to be fixed. I am ready to be reborn. Twenty-one months since my diagnosis, countless trips to the hospital, endless tests and treatments, and now, finally,

I am here. I'm stubborn, perhaps argumentative, and notoriously opinionated, but I am right. If you're a patient who's being asked to carry an unfeasible burden, please, speak up. You don't have to be a physician to advocate for yourself.

THE REALITY CHECK
AND DESCENT

As hard as you think it is, you end up wishing it were that easy.

—EMMA, *TERMS OF ENDEARMENT*

I read the notebook, watch the videos, ask the questions, research, review educational materials, and attend the informational sessions. I sign lengthy consents. I feel informed. I feel prepared. I feel ready. Intellectually and conceptually, I understand, but I really have no actual clue. A stem cell transplant is a journey of incomprehensible suffering, a true test of the limits of human endurance.

The nurse in the video is smiling and has a chatty, upbeat, singsong, preschool-teacher-like delivery. She uses phrases like "a little nausea" and "some mouth pain." The doctor, too, is matter-of-fact and informative as he reviews the side effects and risks on the consent form. There is no emotional overlay, no hint of the brutality you will face. None of this conveys the truth of what will really happen.

I suggest they film a patient too weak to sit vomiting repeatedly into the trash can and screaming in agonized wails. Put *that* in the video. Play *that* for the treatment consent. Their sanitized, smiley, happy face presentation is a load of bologna.

The occupational therapist assesses me as "independent," as in not requiring help with activities of daily living or mobility. She's a tough bird. She tells me, "Remember, you are not here to be sick. You are here to be well."

Wait. What?

I am here to be sick, and if these folks do their jobs, hopefully I'll leave here well. The instant I start trending even a nanometer toward being well, I am out of here. If I were here to just "be well," I would have enrolled in a wellness retreat! I say none of this, but my expression may have given me away.

Here's how this transplant thing will go down: they will wipe out as much of my bone marrow as possible because it is crap. My chemotherapy is to be ablative. Yes, *ablative*. They are *ablating* my existing bone marrow. Destroying it. The chemo will be as strong as it can be. The cancer tries to kill me, the doctors try to kill the cancer, and the process just about kills me. Then the nurses save me.

> A stem cell transplant is a journey of incomprehensible suffering, a true test of the limits of human endurance.

I received test doses of the most toxic chemotherapeutic agent to evaluate my individual metabolism of this drug. Samples were tested at a specialty lab to tweak my personal dosing. Now they can crank up the juice as high as I can withstand without killing me. This process fascinates me. This is not a standard dose; this is *my* dose.

I will receive two ablative chemotherapeutic agents daily over the first four days. It's strong and will *ablate* my bone marrow. To be clear, it's impossible to get rid of every single malignant cell in the bone marrow. That would kill me. The goal is to knock down that marrow as far possible while still keeping me alive. I receive no radiation. Four days of chemo, and then hopefully, no more chemo ever again for as long as I live.

ONCOLOGY 101: TRANSPLANT BIOLOGY SEMINAR NO. 1

Hold on
Hold on to yourself
For this is gonna hurt like hell
—SARAH MCLACHLAN, "HOLD ON"

In the most basic terms, antineoplastic agents, or chemotherapeutic cancer drugs, target rapidly replicating cells. Rapid replication is the hallmark of cancer cells. The super bummer is that the chemotherapy does not limit itself to targeting cancer cells. The chemotherapy is indiscriminate. It targets other healthy, rapidly replicating cells, whether in the skin, hair follicles, gastrointestinal tract, or all the mucous membranes in the body.

I glide across the threshold of my chemo days with the misconception that the side effects will occur roughly chronologically, along the same timeframe as the chemo. I believe that once I push through these four days, I'll be over the first hurdle. Again, wrong.

The nausea starts fairly immediately with the infusions. I am hit with the big blast of it right there on day one, then it lingers, worsens, and sticks around for the long term. The side effects of the chemo come in rolling, overlapping waves of organ decimation and misery.

Initially, I think I'm ahead of the game with chemo. I'd done it before and did well. That must have been some low-grade, weakling, wimpy, itty-bitty, teeny-weeny chemo. This is real, double-black-diamond, supersized slushy chemo, and it major, big-time sucks. Four days of infusions, two drugs. They, too, come in little yellow bags. The nurses check them and hang them up, and then in the poison flows.

"It makes you sick before it makes you well" is a common refrain in oncology. The nausea tsunami is severe, unrelenting, crushing, all-encompassing, and inescapable, with profuse, repetitive vomiting. Trash cans, vomit bags, and toilet—they all fill right up. Each evening the nurse comes right back in with the little yellow bags.

Meanwhile, my emesis bag becomes my security blanket, and I hold on to it tightly for comfort, like a stuffed animal. There are several in the bed and on my nightstand. I do not want to risk barfing on the bed linens, my clothes, or the floor. This kind of vomiting gives no warning, and I am still proud to have never barfed outside of an appropriate receptacle. I tell this to the nurses every time, but they're not impressed.

Why can't my body just chill and accept this stuff? The oncology dietitian explains his caveman theory of nausea: For seven million years of human evolution, purging was our most basic defense against invading toxins, poisons, and pathogens. It gets the gnarly crap out of our systems and has done so for all time. Our body recognizes this chemo as the toxic intruder it is and wants it gone.

I am on four anti-nausea medications. One gives me crazy, vivid dreams, complete with action-packed, high-speed chase scenes and flights across the Grand Canyon in a blue buggy. I have hyperacute sensory overload. Heavy metal music is blaring out of the air vents in the room. I love '80s metal, but this is excessive. I can *clearly* hear Mötley Crüe and Judas Priest being piped into my room. I *know* that it's just an air vent, but I still hear the music blaring out of it. I ask the nurses if they can close off the vent because the music is so loud; it's probably workers on another floor rocking out to some hair bands.

91

The nurses don't even look at me like I am whacked. They know which medication is the culprit, and they stop it. I need sleep and quiet, not crazy dreams and metal music. I know the medical staff is doing everything they can to ease my Barf-O-Rama, but the side effects are outweighing the benefits.

Now I'm down to three anti-nausea medications. I continue to develop acute visual hallucinations. I repeatedly turn my head to look over my right shoulder, where I see an evil little blue creature laughing at me. A nursing student in the room excitedly says she just learned about this in her oncology pharmacology class and knows exactly which medication is causing it. We promptly cut that one out too. The creature recedes forever, and I do not miss it. The two remaining medications do the best they can.

The right regimen of medication is better than no medication, but it's never a rousing win. Every second remains filled with nausea.

> The right regimen of medication is better than no medication, but it's never a rousing win.

It is *the* primary physical and emotive sensation. Mr. Big Green Barf is always in the room. Whatever I push through, they've got more to throw at me. With every gnarly side effect, there are even more coming.

I ask the dietitian and the most experienced oncology nurse how long it will be this bad. The dietitian is crystal clear. "You will have some nausea for sixty to ninety days. Count on it. You will go *home* on nausea medications. It will get progressively better, but prepare for sixty to ninety days."

Okay. That's one answer. I accept it.

Then the nurse responded with her own opinion, after years of dealing with barfing transplant patients. "In my experience you'll be this bad for five days after the last chemo dose. Get through the chemo and the subsequent five days, and it will start to subside a bit."

Humor is everywhere and arises unexpectedly. On one of my sickest days, my eighteen-year-old son calls me from the side of Interstate 70, heading over Vail Pass. He asks me if I can download his proof of insurance and send it to his phone. He's been stopped by a state trooper for expired tags.

He says, "Mom, I was not speeding!" as if he deserves an award. Then he asks if I'd like to speak to the trooper.

I'm in the epicenter of barfdom, confusion, and misery.

"No, I do not wish to speak to the trooper. I gave you the insurance card for your glove box. Why are your tags expired? Do you realize that I'm lying in a hospital bed getting a stem cell transplant and am very sick?"

"Oh, yeah. Sorry, Mom. I hope you feel better. But I really *do* need the insurance, or this guy is not going to let me go."

I open my laptop, download, and send his insurance. He's still on the side of the highway.

"Got it. Thanks, Mom."

Then he's gone.

The lovely cleaning lady, whom by now I know well, is quietly grinning and snickering. "I understand. My son is exactly the same," she says.

Between vomiting and lower gastrointestinal tract explosions, I find vomiting more palatable to describe. Nevertheless, the other circumstance must be addressed. I'll try to keep my description of this passing-of-gastrointestinal-tissue phase mercifully short.

Chemo attacks and damages all fifteen feet of the gastrointestinal tract. In the process the intestine sloughs and passes dead tissue as it loses its absorptive function and the intestine loses fluid. Out flows whatever food has gone in, as well as dead chunks, strips, and slices of intestinal mucosa. If you feel you may need to go to the toilet, do not delay. Do not ponder the situation. *Run.* There is no time.

I initially refused a bedside commode, which was stupid. Just suck it up and realize there may not be time to get to the bathroom. Large, catastrophic, watery releases happen, packed with nasty internal tissue. Your insides are coming out, right into that toilet.

This goes on for days, perhaps weeks, sometimes many times per day. The digestive tract is simply not digesting, and it takes time to heal the gut. Sometimes there may be a reprieve and a rest, but know it's coming back.

ONCOLOGY 101: TRANSPLANT BIOLOGY SEMINAR NO. 2

Down in the waves
She screams again
Roar at the door
My mind can't take much more

—THE BLACK KEYS, "GOLD ON THE CEILING"

After three of my four days receiving the two ablative chemo drugs, I get to start another medication that I lovingly refer to as "the rabbit crap."

Now for a brief science break. Stem cells are smart. They replace stinky bone marrow with good stuff. Stem cells are blood cell precursors and differentiate into three types: red, white, and platelets. The new stem cells set up a blood cell factory, which is called *engrafting* or *engraftment*. The new graft is the blood-cell-producing life source—the real deal, the fountain. I visualize that new cell factory graft as a healthy, colorful, life-springing coral reef in my marrow.

Donor stem cells also bring along T cells, a type of white cell with powerful function. I see them as crazy little ingrate critters zipping around in souped-up sports coupes, wreaking havoc in their path. Some havoc is beneficial, and some is harmful. T cells have the awesome function of recognizing residual cancer cells, which they chomp up and destroy.

Again, ablative chemotherapy does not and cannot kill every single cancer cell because the patient would die as collateral damage. After ablation, there are cancer cells left behind, and the T cells are there to dispose of them. Stem cells are a new marrow factory, and T cells are a potent cancer-fighting therapy, and they take out the lingering malignant freeloaders.

I will be getting a powerful cancer treatment—*nonchemo* cancer treatment—from these T cells. The graft is not only a marrow replacement but also a cancer-fighting treatment, probably the most powerful of all. The system sounds perfect.

However, these cancer ninja T cells tend to get carried away, and they can start attacking their host in addition to the cancerous cells. This is what happens in developing the dreaded GVHD: T cells can perceive the recipient's tissues as foreign, then go on the attack. Even with a good match and a healthy host, unruly T cells can end up having their host for a snack.

I'm not at risk of rejecting the graft; I am at risk of being rejected *by* the graft. It's a double agent. The same thing saving me could attack me. GVHD problems can last forever, for years, or not at all. Meanwhile, I'm in denial that I might get it. I simply do not want to go there. I'm resigned that if I get it, I get it and will be a pawn in its toaster forever.

Meanwhile, the doctors put considerable energy into preventing it. Transplant recipients receive immunosuppressive medications to neutralize some T cells to prevent GHVD. I have two immunosuppressives already planned for my regimen. Dr. Good Ideas wants to be aggressive and add a third GVHD prevention: the rabbit.

Rabbit antithymocyte globulin (rabbit ATG) is an intravenous biologic given before the transplant. It sticks around to clear out T cells as they come swimming in with the stem cells, and it must be given in advance.

"What's the big deal?" I ask. "Sounds like we should do this."

"It can be hard to tolerate. It has side effects. You may get a fever and chills," advised Dr. Good Ideas.

No biggie. I'm in. Hook me up.

"The night of the rabbit" was perhaps the most dramatic of this entire journey; I was completely incapacitated. "Fever and chills" was an understatement. I wish I could remember my primary nurse's name from that night. I can still picture her and hear her voice. I know she never left my bedside, never stopped working, moving, thinking, and acting. If there were a consummate training film for exemplary nursing care in critical situations, it was her. The nurse was a wizard—a brilliant, knowledgeable, experienced, calm, unflappable wizard.

I spend much of my career reassuring my patients that they do not need to panic about fevers. For the most part, they're a natural part of an illness. We generally need to move away from the culture of fever phobia. Patients may be treated for *comfort*, but not all fevers need to be *treated*. We need to look at the whole picture of the patient's illness.[1] This rabbit potion, however, caused the kind of high fever that my oncology team did *not* want. This kind of fever can be dangerous, hard to manage, and can cycle upward.

I also got rigors, a word that's tossed around a lot in medical lingo. I'd always thought of them as bad chills. Let me tell you, these were more than bad chills. These were uncontrollable, shaking chills, coupled with muscle spasms that utterly take control of your body. Needless to say, it was a rough night. Someone gave me a warm blanket for the chills, and I cuddled beneath it.

---

1   This is not specific case-based medical advice. Please always contact your provider or your child's provider for any specific instance of illness for personalized attention, with or without fever. Immunosuppressed patients, however, *do* need to act promptly with fevers. Potentially dangerous fevers can be seen with such events as being locked in a hot car or from an anesthesia reaction in susceptible patients.

Then my fever spiked higher and higher. The wizard nurse told me, "We have to bring this down." They drew blood cultures to look for sepsis, then immediately administered antibiotics. They gave me an intravenous dose of an opiate narcotic medication for the rigors and to help stop the spasms. Then the nurse looked at me and said, "We're going to pack you on ice like a fish."

As I struggled to ask how that would be possible, I was immediately packed on ice like a halibut in a market. Instantly, several nurses placed ice packs under my head, back, and legs; in my armpits; and on top of me. My primary nurse and all of her assistants were completely calm and betrayed no panic or anxiety, only professionalism and action. I never for a second doubted their expertise and skill.

My blood pressure plummeted, and I received IV fluid boluses and who knows what else. My fever came down. The rigors dissipated, and as bonus I stopped vomiting. I believe the episode lasted about two hours.

The rabbit infusion continued, and I survived. At some point during the night, I achieved a normal body temperature, and in the morning, I awoke to the light of day.

ONCOLOGY NURSES

I can tell a new story now ...
Surely then
See the curtain rising to show us once again
All the magic of the earth and the skies
See the more we find
The more we realize ...
High above
High above
So sure inspired again

—YES, "HOLY LAMB"

Oncology nurses are a special breed. I have an equal number of male and female oncology nurses over the course of my stay, and each one is amazing. They're nurturing. They care. They have so much experience, specifically on the bone marrow transplant unit. They inspire confidence. Your life is in their hands, and they cannot mess up—not a dosage, a medication, a rate of flow, an assessment, a moment of monitoring, or a concerning symptom. They cannot miss *anything*, and they do not. Nothing is too much for them. They know what to do and how to do it quickly. Their calm demeanor is pervasive and provides a sense of trust. I never doubt them for a millisecond.

Do not try to argue with an oncology nurse. You will lose. They're polite too; you won't even realize that you were owned until they leave.

Adequate superlatives for these people escape me. I respect them so much that I never wanted one to have to clean up my barf.

Later I needed a shower but was not able to stand safely. My blood pressure was dangerously low, so I was a major fall risk. I told my deeply caring male nurse that I didn't want to be too old-fashioned but that I preferred a female aide for the shower. Not to insult or question his professionalism or anything, but he was not going anywhere *near* my shower. He laughed and said that I *was* old-fashioned and that he'd have a female aide there to help within three minutes.

I'll never forget them ripping off my toasty blanket and packing me on ice for as long as I live. I was laughing about it with the nurses by the next morning. "When you said you were going to pack me on ice, I didn't even know what you meant, and then presto chango, I was on ice. It was like something out of *Bewitched*."

THE DONOR

What can I give you in return?

—LULU, "TO SIR WITH LOVE"

I staged a statistical coup in that both of my sisters were perfect donor matches. Moreover, they both offered their stem cells to me without question or reservation. My older sister, Donna, has grown children, a happily retired husband, and the freedom to work remotely, thanks to COVID-19, so I chose her because it was less disruptive to her family.

She was fully on board and willing to do whatever they asked to save my life. No fear, no complaints, no hesitation, no burden. She could have donated in New York but made the choice to come to Colorado. She had her entire workup here and was able to directly deliver her cells to me from the clinic next to the hospital. After a comprehensive medical evaluation, she received a squeaky-clean bill of health.

I saw her briefly in the clinic, and she came to see me after my pretransplant bone marrow biopsy, but for the most part, we were relegated to the parallel universes of donor and recipient. I know we spoke during my four chemo days in the hospital, but my recollection of that is minimal to nonexistent. Most of the details here come from her.

First, when she came to the clinic for her screening labs, a nurse entered her room carrying a gargantuan trash bag of blood-drawing tubes. My sister innocently assumed that she was organizing all those tubes for all of her patients for the entire day. Nope. They were all for her.

Next was the venous access assessment. My sister is tough as nails and has not a squeamish bone in her body, but this was her first harvest. Yes, indeed, she was there to be *harvested*.

In one of my educational videos, the recipient is cautioned that they should view the donor as a human and not just a donor. I find this hilarious, as I had totally slipped into that mindset. In my mind my sister had become a petri dish of my new cells—a vessel. I had completely dehumanized her. Oops! Sorry, Donna!

To assess her vein integrity, they use tourniquets to repeatedly check her veins. They tap, pat, rub, and distress them, all the while talking about their quality. "Look at these. These look good. Then that one. We can get a large IV into that one. Ah, *this* one looks good too."

She notices the room is beginning to spin. She feels hot, then cold, then woozy and shaky. As she's about to hit the deck, she asks for a cool neckcloth, and if possible, could they please do what they need to do without talking about her veins and lines? "Oh," they say, "sorry. We didn't think about that." She took a break and got some water, and the nurses quietly figured out the whole vein deal out of earshot.

> While the terms "bone marrow transplant" and "stem cell transplant" are often used interchangeably, the latter is more accurate and current.

Next, they want to show her their stem cell extraction machine. She can clearly see how proud they are of their nifty machine and does not want to hurt their feelings but politely declines. In any case she'll see plenty of it on donation day.

While the terms "bone marrow transplant" and "stem cell transplant" are often used interchangeably, the latter is more accurate and current. Nowadays bone marrow isn't taken directly from the donor. Dr. Good Ideas explained that they get *more* stem cells by harvesting them from the peripheral bloodstream.

Because I'll be needing a cool five million stem cells, my sister receives a few days' worth of injections to stimulate production. Her bones ache as marrow chugs away, producing my new stem cells. Ibuprofen and extra sleep are the tickets.

Then after five weeks in Colorado for her medical evaluation, two COVID-19 tests, observation for symptoms, and round of injections, the day has finally come: harvest day.

She gets her two intravenous lines in silence. They pull her blood from a large-bore intravenous line in one site and run it through a fancy-schmancy machine that circulates her entire blood volume *six times*. Once her blood has been stripped of stem cells, the machine returns the blood to her through another large-bore line in her other arm. This process takes about seven hours.

They needed five million stem cells, and she made seven million. *Way* more than needed. She's always been a pathological overachiever. They ultimately gave me six million; we have a million in surplus if I ever need a stem cell booster in the future.

My husband picks her up. She's exhausted from the process and the premedication. She demolishes a hamburger, takes a nice snooze, and flies home two days later. Donor out. I really needed those cells. Thanks for saving my life.

MY BRIGHT RED CELLS

And we can force you to be free
And we can force you to believe
And I close my eyes and tighten up my brain ...
I will fight for the right to be right ...
And I want to believe
That a light's shining through
Somehow ...
I want to live

—DAVID BOWIE, "CYGNET COMMITTEE"

Time of day: Unknown. Nighttime? I think so. I *think* it's dark outside; there's no orange glow. After rabbit day two and chemo day four, I get my new cells. I have irrational fears and ask the nurse how we know they won't be dropped or mistakenly go to someone else. Apparently, this is common.

Two people carry them in a cooler. They are neatly labeled, checked, and rechecked several times by two separate nurses. As my sister finishes her donation, her cells are walked up to me right then and there, then administered straight from her infusion bag directly into my bloodstream via my central line. This next part blows me away. Hang on to your new age science book: the cells know exactly where to go. They travel from the bloodstream to the bone marrow space. They are self-starters. No instruction manual needed. The cells know where to go.

I have a picture burned permanently into my brain of my bag of bright-red stem cells. I fought so hard and waited so long for them, and now here they are. I put my sister through so much. I put my family through so much. I have negotiated with so many doctors. I have pleaded for my life, and now here it is, in a bag of bright-red cells.

I am so grateful to the doctors, scientists, patients who have come before me—the people who came up with the idea, were brave enough to try it, patient enough to study, perfect, and improve it. I am also grateful to Dr. Good Ideas, the doctor of grandness of thought and economy of words, who agreed to proceed.

The cells go in. It's the first moment of the rest of my life.

The next few days are a cloud of nausea and vomiting. It's a learning moment. I thought the chemo barf was done, or at least about to wind down, but the delayed chemo effect can be worse than the immediate effect. I recall the smart nurse who said there would be five severe days after the last chemo day. Okay. I like having a number, and she was right. After five days, the vomiting goes from relentless to scattered.

In the meantime I develop a debilitating headache. It feels like an ice pick in my brain. This isn't a typical side effect, and I'm not sure if I should just deal or talk about it with my providers. Here, I learned something important: in this unit, they take *everything* seriously. They want and need to know, and they've probably heard it before. They truly know how you feel.

> I put my sister through so much. I put my family through so much. I have negotiated with so many doctors. I have pleaded for my life, and now here it is, in a bag of bright-red cells.

105

If you have a symptom, tell the staff. They will move mountains to get to the bottom of it and help. When I tell them about the headache, they suspect it's a medication reaction, go through my list, and switch a few things around.

My in-house oncologist at this time is an Italian doctor. We'll call him Dr. Italian. He is brilliant, kind, and old school. I'm doing well if I can understand one out of every six words he says, but I can read his gesticulations to fill in the gaps. He makes me feel that I'm his only patient. He always sits in the room, never seems rushed, and gives his pure focus and time. He is thorough. He is experienced. He is not just "doing his rounds." He is *my* doctor.

I am not at all confident that the magic headache cure exists in his bag of tricks, but while they figure it out, I make some changes of my own. I realize that I'm under a high level of electronic and communication stress in the unit. I have three electronic devices in my bed alone. Any glance at a screen makes my headache scream. I put them all aside.

Family and friends of transplant patients are worried every second, and they want information. They call, text, and email constantly. Giving updates regarding each symptom, treatment, and progress report; detailing the ups and downs; and reliving the pain cause extreme stress and take up time best spent resting. Good news can bring misplaced relief and idealism, and bad news is seen as a major setback, even though it's all part of the process.

Personally, I feel overwhelmed and guilty every time I report a negative symptom, and presently, there are *only* negative symptoms. Instead, I comfort and reassure my friends and family. We have no information as to whether the transplant is working—yet. We have nothing but severe but fully expected side effects.

I decide to suspend all communication, cut everyone off except for my husband, and stop looking at screens entirely. This saves my sanity, and no one takes offense. I need to rest, period. Everyone understands. As my husband becomes command central, even my interactions with him are brief. The effort to sit up and merely hold a device is excruciating. I have the nurse call my husband when I cannot. I do not want my husband, kids, friends, or family to hear me this beaten down anyway. The headache affects my sensorium to the extent that I am not myself.

Dr. Italian decides upon a treatment plan, orders a medication for the headache, and alters some of my other medications. I do not know what he prescribes; for all I know, it may be Sicilian jellyfish extract. I just know that it knocks me out and kills that headache. I think I lose about two days, then we ease off. Four days or so later, the headache is gone.

> Tell your caretakers everything. It can be the difference between life and death.

Next, I have an episode of mild tenderness and swelling over the insertion of my central line. Again, it may be nothing, and I do not want to be dramatic, but I mention it. The doctor immediately starts five days of IV antibiotics for central line infection. The pain and swelling go away. It's a good thing I told them, as this is how line infections start. Again, I'm trying to drive a point home: tell your caretakers *everything*. It can be the difference between life and death. We are *the* sickest, highest-risk patients in the hospital. Report every symptom.

RUDE FOOD AWAKENING

You don't look very well. Are you sure it wasn't that gray
kind of lamb, or you ate a lot of that weird chicken?
I think you'd just feel better if you threw up.

—HELEN, *BRIDESMAIDS*

When I awake from the headache haze, I have a day of hunger.
It's a welcome feeling; I have not felt hungry in a while. I
want a sandwich. The nurses are willing to take a credit card to get
their patients real food from the lobby food carts. I insist they buy
themselves a real food item and always leave a generous tip.

Unfortunately, I have a severe aversion to the cafeteria food. I
order a breakfast burrito one morning, and the pale, shriveled jalapeño
that accompanies it looks like a diseased gallbladder on my plate.
Disgusting. I cannot even look at the *tray* from the cafeteria. The best
I can hope for is a fruit smoothie in a cup. To this day I *still* can't even
think about that tray—immediate heaving.

When my real sandwich comes up, it looks good, and I take a
bite. Slimy, mealy, tasteless mush. Awful texture. Sand, slop, paste,
swill. No detectable flavor. I spit it out, and the rest goes in the trash.
I now have an immediate aversion to all sandwiches, and one by one,
foods turn from positive memories to aversions. I know how that
sandwich is *supposed* to taste. Now all I perceive is horrible, gross,
inedible. This is my new normal. My taste buds are gone.

My tongue is full of ridges, peeling tissue, and missing strips. Even something as basic as lemon-lime soda tastes like a cleaning chemical. I am down to applesauce, crackers, juice, and fruit smoothies. Each of these, over time, eventually comes up and into the trash can. The hunger snap quickly ends. I want nothing. Food is not what it used to be. Things that I loved are replaced by intense aversions. It sucks.

My grandiose plans of bed exercises and walking the hallway never happened. What a joke! I lie in that bed and barely move unless I absolutely must. I barely turn my head for fear of triggering vomiting. I rarely sit up, except to attempt to eat, drink, or lean over the trash can or emesis bag.

Now Dr. Italian is back to see me. We discuss my Sicilian grand-mother's desserts—*struffoli, sfinci, crostoli*—and he corrects my pro-nunciation. He has a style of warning the patient before complications arrive. He says he doesn't wish to create more anxiety for me but that it's good to know what to expect. He's on the right track. I want to know everything in store for me.

I was briefly convinced that I was done with the hard part. Not so fast. Dr. Italian does not want to burst my bubble but warns that mucositis is next. My mouth feels crazy weird, but I have no pain.

"This will change," he says. "It will flare within twenty-four hours. It can be severe. When it does, please ask for pain medication right away." After a pause, he added, "It is barbaric what we do to you patients. Absolutely barbaric."

He says this with genuine compassion, and it is strangely com-forting to hear. I already agree, and I've not even been as deep as I am going to go in this cave of horrors. It makes one wonder how much the human body can endure. How do the older patients survive?

Dr. Italian also wants to discuss upcoming changes to my skin. He's found that patients deal with it better if they are warned. Okay, let's have it, pal.

"One of your chemo agents will cause you to have thick, dry, dark brown skin after a few weeks. It can be distressing, but it should be expected. It will not last forever, and it is not serious, but it *can* last for a few weeks. It is preferable that you know. It may be all over—face, chest, arms, legs, back. You will develop a deep, dark tan, your skin will become rough, and then it will flake and peel off."

I'm sold. At least it doesn't sound painful. This gives me something to look forward to. I am so grateful to Dr. Italian for just putting everything on the table. Propped up and empowered by intense denial, I'm ever hopeful that I will skip right over this little mouth sore problem.

Then it hits: raw, open, burning wounds take over my mouth.

> I find relief in it being me here in this room and not any of my other loved ones.

Ulcers, strips of raw burning flesh, and chemical burns cover my inner cheeks, tongue, throat, and esophagus. And there's still nausea and vomiting to boot. At the peak, I scream out loud with each excruciating swallow.

Patients need to be prepared for this agony. I have mouthwashes, coating medications, and topical anesthetics, and they help but only briefly. They give me two different opiate pain medications via three different delivery systems: intravenous, oral, and patch.

Profuse vomiting returns, then ramps up to new extremes. I am not meant for these opiates. Vomiting over open sores is indescribable agony. They offer me more and different opiates, and I decline. They offer suction for secretions, which sounds unpleasant, so I decline that too.

I spend six long days in this phase and push through. I never want to go through this again. There are patients who have had more than one stem cell transplant. They must be tough beyond tough. I do not know how older or sicker patients endure and cannot conceive of a child being in my shoes.

I find relief in it being *me* here in this room and not any of my other loved ones. I hope it will provide positive karma for them. It's too horrible to think of anyone else in this position, and I'm so relieved they cannot visit. I want no one to see me like this, besides the medical staff. I particularly cannot imagine my husband seeing me in this much pain. He senses it through my voice, though I can barely speak. He knows, and he feels it. He does not need to see it.

SLOUGHING TISSUE

More than this
You know there's nothing
−ROXY MUSIC, "MORE THAN THIS"

The body I walked in with has truly been left behind. I'm reminiscent of my medical school cadaver. My skin and nails are waxy, plasticky, yellowish, friable, and soft. I feel synthetic. My nose has mucosal tissue curtains. My mouth is all over the place, barely attached. It feels not only nonfunctional but also nonpresent—mealy, ridged, peeling, and gross. My mouth does not have the taste function and does not detect textures, and it's hard to chew. For now, I am a plastic person.

My body is not my own, and I feel like I am about to fall apart in the bed. My fingernails develop a brownish-maroon elevated band at the base of the nail. It looks like a discolored frost heave in a northern road. As it grows out, I can start to see a new, healthy nail coming in behind it. I call it "the chemo band." I am not sure what it's *actually* called, but it is certainly ugly. They tell me it will grow out in two to three months.

The tissue is coming off in slices, slivers, and chunks. It forms curtains in my nose. You're not supposed to attempt to remove it in any forceful way; gently blowing one's nose in the shower is the key. Some will come out when moist, only to build up again. My mouth is crumbly and coarse with loose, hanging mucosal tissues. I feel them schlepping down my throat.

It's so hard to eat anything. Most of my protein intake comes from digesting my own oral tissues. I can feel a hole on the underside of my tongue and at the back of my throat. The throat sucker is the worst. I moan. I writhe. I clench. I scream. The dietitian comes in again and asks how I'm doing.

"Anything that comes at me causes nausea, vomiting, abdominal cramping, and diarrhea. It hurts to swallow anything. I can barely take in an ounce or a bite."

"Well, you've got to keep eating."

He explains that if I fail to use my gut, it sits dormant. I picture my intestine as a useless, flaccid, decaying, mucosal eel. But it's also a sitting target. If it's not taken out for an occasional walk, the tissue is perceived as dead by the vulturous T cells. If they attack, I may get gastrointestinal GVHD.

Okay, pass the hot wings. I try to consume whatever tiny sips and bites that I can. Everyone's suggestions end up in the trash can: the crackers, the potatoes, the smoothies, the applesauce. I remain on a steady diet of agonizing pain. I feel guilt and failure from my unsuccessful attempts at enteric nourishment, but I know that I'm trying.

ABSOLUTE NEUTROPHIL COUNT (ANC): TRANSPLANT BIOLOGY SEMINAR NO. 3

I have met my destiny in quite a similar way
The history book on the shelf
Is always repeating itself

—ABBA, "WATERLOO"

Absolute neutrophil count (ANC) is a big deal in blood cancers and critical for so many reasons. The neutrophil is the most common type of white blood cell, the first line of defense for bacterial, viral, and fungal infections, and is in charge of locating and healing damaged tissue. The ANC is how these healer neutrophils are measured and reported, and every patient knows they won't feel better until they appear.

The oncology nurses know the ANC will appear and rise. They've seen it time and again, playing out in the unit like a never-ending rerun. The oncology nurse writes my daily ANC on the whiteboard in my room every morning. It's a big moment. Transplant recipients watch this number as if their life depends upon it because it does.

The appearance of a rising ANC shows that you are engrafting, and it heralds when you will start to heal your sores and come out of the dark days of pure hell. They repeatedly tell you to be patient and wait for days ten to fourteen posttransplant, when the ANC starts to appear. It tends to start low, then there's a big increase. The anticipation is excruciating. Watching that nurse write my number on the board is burned into my mind. The lowest ANC that I register is 10, and a normal count is in the 1,500 to 6,000 range. Ouch.

My level of exhaustion is still extreme. Getting out of bed for a shower or the bathroom still requires assistance. In my former life as a physically strong human, I completed a full-distance, off-road triathlon. Before I became a fragile, vomiting shell, my husband and I completed a thirty-eight-mile day—twelve-mile bike approach, twenty-one-mile hike, and five-mile finisher hike. I thought *that* was a big day. It has nothing on the exhaustion caused by this transplant.

Day twelve: ANC 40. Extremely low but up from 10. I'm making neutrophils. Day sixteen: 89.

The nurse says, "We see healing at 200. You may start to notice this later today." Can it be true? Maybe.

Later that day, I feel my first pang of relief. Slightly less screaming. The deepest of my esophageal pain subsides. The graft is taking root.

Day seventeen: ANC 650. I can start to see the sun again. I am out of the extreme sepsis danger zone. I feel the pain lifting. My wounds continue to improve.

Day nineteen: ANC 2,779. I am officially out of hell. My last, most evil sore is healing well. My husband is not an excessively emotive individual, but I can hear him beaming through the phone.

I believed my nurses and doctors and shared their faith that my ANC would increase. But I would not be fully convinced until I saw it on that whiteboard. I was in the depth of sickness when I opened my eyes and saw the nurse write "40." At that moment, I knew I had engraftment and that eventually I would get to go home.

The staff encourages me to get up out of bed and walk to prepare. I have been bedridden for a month. I intentionally get up and walk the halls during rounds so all the mean doctors can see me.

One of my new in-patient doctors, Dr. Believer, specializes in Waldenström's lymphoma and takes special interest in my case. He, too, wants to know why it took almost two years for me to get a transplant and is especially curious about my quality of life during the infamous three months where I felt better after my first treatment round. We discuss those months at length. I tell him about the short rides, the short walks, and the slow jogs.

> I know with 100 percent certainty that no matter what complications may arise and whatever future struggles I endure, this is the smartest thing I ever pushed for in my life.

Dr. Believer asks if I was satisfied living like that. "It was better than feeling sick all the time. I thought I'd be able to build up stamina. Then it became clear the illness was taking over again. For a time, yes, I thought that that could be my new life. It was certainly better than what I had before any treatment."

"Did I hear that you are a biker?"

"Yes, I am. Or I was."

He looks at me with a thoughtful, astonished doctor face and says, "Carol, that level of activity and function was never going to be good enough for you. It was not an adequate response. There was no reason to even *consider* accepting that quality of life. I'm glad you pushed for your transplant."

This wonderful doctor was right.

I do not regret any of the steps I took to get here, but my relief at being here and not living in a diminished state is immeasurable. I know with 100 percent certainty that no matter what complications may arise and whatever future struggles I endure, this is the smartest thing I ever pushed for in my life.

Stem cell transplants for MDS are effective, accepted, evidence based, validated, and trusted. Transplants for Waldenström's, on the other hand, are relatively new, but they have been done. There is some medical literature but not a lot of patients or outcome data. It can be considered experimental, but Dr. Believer is full of positivity for my cure. I cling to his opinion, as I have with so many others along the way.

REFLECTIONS ON SURVIVAL

Never been a time where there was a fork in my road.

—FRANK, *WILD*

A psychologist, Dr. Warm and Fuzzy, visits me in my hospital room from time to time. She says she has stopped by many times, but I was either asleep, unconscious, or unable to talk to her. I hope she did not take offense. During that period of severe mouth sores, I rarely spoke.

She asks me how I get through. She asks the same of every patient. She wants to share insight and coping skills for the benefit of future patients.

I tell her that I get through based on commitment to a few specific beliefs. One is complete trust that this was the only thing that I could do to live. There was no fork in my road. No matter what happens, this transplant was the only thing that could give me another shot at a normal life. If I get GVHD, or if I die, this is *still* what I would've done. I will never look back. I have no regrets.

> My unshakable belief and trust in the medical and nursing care here also provides tremendous solace.

My unshakable belief and trust in the medical and nursing care here also provides tremendous solace. I am completely comfortable in the hands of this staff. I trust the science, the process, the knowledge, and the humans delivering this care; I trust it all. Someone with a distrust of the medical profession, hospitals, or science would have a much harder time when scary things start happening. I know that in the hands of these nurses, I am safe.

The big picture of how to get through? Easy. Gratitude and positivity. Positivity will not cure you, but it helps you from moment to moment. Moreover, I have gratitude for so many things: I have lived a full life. I have no regrets. I have done all I need to do. Lack of regret makes way for gratitude. I tell her how relieved I am to be getting this done now, before I'm older, sicker, or weaker. With each unfortunate episode of deep physical pain and torture, I still know it won't last forever.

I'm also grateful that I have health insurance and that I will not be going bankrupt from cancer. I own my business, so I will not be fired because of cancer either. These are terrifying realities for so many people who risk losing their jobs, their insurance, their credit, or their homes all because of cancer.

I'm grateful that my kids are older and that they can live their lives without depending on me to care for them. They have their father. I am grateful that my husband can care for me and continue to work full-time remotely. Despite cancer and COVID-19, we're surviving. I am guilt-ridden because I'm not working, even if that's outside of my control.

I'm grateful that my parents are alive into their nineties and living to see me get this transplant. I am grateful for all the brave patients who have come before me. I'm grateful that I was able to spend time with my family before entering the hospital. Through illness, lockdowns, and not being able to work, I always found something to do, whether writing, learning to bake, walking outside, or hanging out with my dogs and my family.

There are depressing days, but they do not last. I have not had a solid wallow of more than twenty-four hours since my initial diagnosis. I seek humor in every situation wherever possible. I put pressure on myself to do everything I am told to the letter, as if that karma of rule-following will make my transplant a success.

There are times when I feel like a burden to my family, and I wonder if I should be putting them through this, especially if the transplant isn't successful. I question whether it would be preferable for my family if I died so they could move on.

It takes a lot of energy to feel sad, useless, and defeated. So when I'm depressed or feeling burdensome, even when feeling waves of suicidality at occasional low points, I combine those dysfunctional psychological responses with my love of true crime. There's always solace in the fact that when you're a depressed, suicidal cancer patient, you have much less fear of serial killers. Here, serial killers can't touch me. I want to see one hooded in a dark alley and tell him, "Forget it, dude. I have been through a stem cell transplant, and you cannot hurt me. You got nothing." Suicidal cancer patients do not mind serial killers. Plus, my family would get my life insurance.

I'm grateful I had the persistence and stamina for self-advocacy. I simply would not let it drop. I am not intimidated by medical professionals. Maybe this is because I'm a physician, and maybe it's my generally pushy personality. If Dr. Good Ideas had not agreed to move forward with this, I would have proceeded to yet another center and then out of state. Any patient can self-advocate; it's not necessary to be a physician or other medical professional.

I am beyond grateful that I have a match and a backup match. Statistics have not otherwise been in my favor. The odds of having both of these rare cancers are infinitesimal. Most doctors believe that

I am purely the victim of unfortunate statistics. Either way, I stopped agonizing over this a long time ago.

Not everyone survives their transplant. Cancer social media gives us access to others' stories, both hopeful and harrowing. One such story is about a young woman with three young sons and an aggressive leukemia. She was adopted and of mixed ethnicity, so it took a long time for her to find her match through the registry. She underwent six rounds of aggressive chemo while waiting; multiply what I went through by *six*. She got her transplant and was officially leukemia-free, then died of a brain bleed and pulmonary fungal infection. The risks are real.

Every time I take a preventive medication, I am thankful for the problems that I do not have and the potential complications that are not being realized. I robotically take so many medications because I know that I'm preventing fungal, bacterial, and viral infections; liver damage; electrolyte abnormalities; vitamin deficiencies; and so much more.

The day I entered the hospital, my husband gave me some devastating news: a dear friend, ten years younger than I, died that same day of chronic alcoholism. For reasons I'll never comprehend, she nurtured her disease rather than herself, and she died. I would rather have cancer than alcoholism. I believe it is more curable.

We had previously talked about our illnesses and how we each wanted to see the other survive, and I will miss her forever. When I have my head in the trash can while barfing up my applesauce or when I can't swallow without yelping in pain, I can still feel that I'm alive and that I'm lucky.

This may have been a longer answer than Dr. Warm and Fuzzy expected, but she takes it all in. When I finish, I look around the room, unaware of how exactly long I'd been speaking. Two nurses and that gem of a cleaning lady are now also standing there, still as statues, looking right at me. Apparently, they'd listened to every word.

TRYING TO GET THE HECK OUT OF HERE

'Cause I've seen blue skies through the tears
In my eyes
And I realize, I'm going home
—TIM CURRY, "I'M GOING HOME"

A physician's assistant tells me that if I can consume a thousand calories and one liter of fluid in a twenty-four-hour period without vomiting, I get to go home. Meanwhile, I'm struggling to consume two hundred calories *per day*.

I tell them I can do better at home in my house with my food, my family, and my dogs, as everything that comes up from food service causes an immediate, intense aversion. I cannot even *look* at it. I've continued to survive on their smoothies, and I don't particularly want to see them anymore either. My room in this hospital causes aversions; simply looking around conjures images of barfing and pain. I gotta get out of here.

The staff has heard all of this before. The no-mess-around physician's assistant points out that if I go home too early, I will be back.

Oh, no. I will *never* be back. This is a one-and-done deal. I will not fail at home. I tell him that I'm quite motivated.

To this the physician's assistant says, "Everyone says that. We hear it all the time."

122

I like this physician's assistant. He's a straight talker.

My futile negotiations continue. "Perhaps that's because everyone *will* do better at home?"

I'm not even close to the calorie or fluid minimum. I'll be going home on daily intravenous fluids, so at least the pressure's off there. I successfully arbitrate a conditional release program of no vomiting for twelve hours and one meal of decent food, including a protein. Then I bribe my nurse to get me a real turkey sandwich from a real sandwich shop and tell them to order whatever they want and to tip the server. I eat the turkey out of the sandwich and do not barf it up. I get to go home!

It will be a shocker for my husband to see me: bald, frail, sickly, pale. My huge head covering completes the look.

> They do not care that I'm bald, frail, and look 115 years old. I am home.

Classic cancer patient chic. My nurse wheels me down to my husband and our Jeep waiting outside.

"You look about 115 years old," he says.

Thanks, sweetie. Spot-on. That's exactly how I feel.

My month in the spa is done. The "long days, short month" cliché applies.

Exactly four weeks ago, I walked wide-eyed into this place. Now I have my new cells, and I am walking out. Piece of cake.

When we get home, the dogs are ecstatic. My husband and kids are equally delighted to have me. Even the cat seems happy. They do not care that I'm bald, frail, and look 115 years old. I am home.

PART III
RECOVERY, LIFE RETRIEVAL, AND BODILY RESTORATION

POSTTRANSPLANT HOME RECOVERY

I'm on my way
Just set me free
Home sweet home

—MÖTLEY CRÜE, "HOME SWEET HOME"

The first few days at home are hard, but there's so much to be thankful for. After all, I'm not dead.

I have a mealy, nasty, gross, sloughing mouth, but at least it doesn't hurt. I can only walk a few yards, but I'm mobile. I can even perform all my own self-care. Everything I manage to eat is going straight to the growth and health of the grafted transplant that's growing stem cells in my marrow. It alone is consuming about three thousand calories per day. My entire metabolism is quite literally focused on that graft, and it's positively sucking me dry. I've lost muscle mass, and my food intake is not going to rebuild those muscles yet. At first I am lucky to eat a few hundred calories per day.

I have a lot of clinic visits, twice per week at first. Blood draw, monitoring, GVHD screening. No driving allowed. My husband takes me to each appointment, and I go nowhere else.

In this initial posttransplant phase, self-care is a full-time job. There's still weakness, fogginess, fatigue, craploads of medication, central line care, IV fluids, line flushes, obsessive cleanliness, a lot of rest, and a preposterous amount of sitting. Our house is small. The walk from our bedroom to the laundry room is very short, and I need to sit down as soon as I complete it, right on top of the clothes in the laundry basket. I quickly learn that if all I can do is walk down the hall, then that is what I will do.

I also learn that I need a chair in which to plop myself down in each and every room. I try to not lie down in bed unless I absolutely must and make an effort to sit in more communal areas. My husband puts a comfortable chair by the front door so I can be part of comings and goings.

In the hospital there was a whole lot going on all the time. Now there's a whole lotta nothing going on. The level of weakness, fatigue, and cognitive drag is dramatic. I need to break down every task into the smallest possible steps. Oral care is not oral care; I need

> In this initial posttransplant phase, self-care is a full-time job.

to perform toothbrushing, flossing, tongue brushing, and mouth rinsing. Four separate steps.

My reaction time is slow. The no-driving rule makes sense. I'm not on any sedating medications, but the cognitive impairment is significant, presumably from the draining, traumatic experience. I know I'd put certain things in certain places before I left so I could find everything easily, but now I can't remember where I put anything.

I can't remember simple words. I'm trying to recall the word "carabiner," a basic piece of climbing gear, and the word is simply gone. I try to explain that I'm looking for "the metal climbing thingy with the pushy-innie gate dealy." I want to use it to hang up my sun hat. No sun allowed; it can cause GVHD of the skin. My son looks at me and says, "Mom. Carabiner." Right, that's it.

Little by little the memory slots fill back up like index cards in an old library catalog. My memories eventually speed up too. It seems like every time I ask how long something will last, the answer is sixty to ninety days.

The transplant team does not want germ exposure from dirty dishes, dirty laundry, the litter box, trash, or any other housework, and I'm too weak and nauseated to perform these functions anyway. Cooking is too dangerous in terms of potential minor trauma, and besides, the smells are nauseating.

I duly adjust my expectations of house management. If clean dishes are available, all four humans and three animals have been fed, the house does not smell, and clean clothes are being worn by all, that counts as a resounding success. Feeling unhelpful around the house is a hard adjustment. When does all this start to get better? When can I do more? Ah, yes, around sixty to ninety days.

I dread the home IV fluids. I initially had visions of the pole, hanging bags, and complicated tubing in my living room for all to see. Mercifully, my worries were misplaced. Technology has made it easy; the fluid comes in a softball-sized container with a tiny internal pump and fits in a little fanny pack. My nurse does a virtual orientation via FaceTime: flush the line, hook up the tube, and the fluid and magnesium infuse over the span of a few hours. At first I mostly sit during this process, but as I get stronger, I can walk around and do things while getting an infusion. Welcome to the future.

My daily shower is a big deal. Getting in and out is taxing. For the first month, I have to sit down the entire time. The fear of falling is real and persistent. Active days mean longer recovery. I walk in the yard with my husband behind me to make sure I do not fall. My muscles are still weak, and my coordination is poor.

But slowly my cognition clears. The magic ninety-day time frame is right on point. Over time I notice significant improvements in my recall, information processing, sequencing, problem-solving ability, and general clarity of thought. Thankfully, my brain is not permanently damaged, and it seems to be bouncing back faster than my guts or hair.

All in all, it's a slog—one slow day after another—yet I only vomit once. Afterward, my husband is clear. "If you vomit again, we're going to the hospital." I take my nausea medication and lie still. I do not vomit again. I am never returning to that hospital.

The most obvious question—the question—continues to creep in and out of my consciousness. Do I still have cancer? My sudden awareness of the lack of cancer symptoms startles me; I do not have leg or back aches or the cancer-sick feeling or feel feverish or flu-like. For two years I have lived with pain and every kind of aching imaginable: body aches, leg aches, back aches, sick cancer aches, muscles aches, bone aches.

I have transplant recovery symptoms but no cancer symptoms. Thinking back, I haven't felt cancer symptoms since about halfway through my hospital stay. They dissipated as the treatment side effects took over. As I'm sitting in the front foyer in my "recovery chair" watching the comings and goings, these realizations hit me like a massive clanging bell. I have no cancer symptoms!

I wasn't sure if I'd ever live without aching because I wasn't sure if I'd ever get that transplant. This is what I've wanted since well before my diagnosis: just getting rid of those damn leg aches. Now they are gone. Did I mention that I have no cancer symptoms? Hopefully, this also means I have no cancer.

ITCHY ZOMBIE

As Dr. Italian warned me, my skin gradually turns dark brown, dry, and scaly. There are simultaneous iguana, alligator, dinosaur, razorback, and leather situations happening, along with various thick, bumpy, cobblestone-like regions. The itching is extraordinary, poison-ivy-like. At night I focus on a spot and scratch and scratch until the area is raw and excoriated; such a bad plan. When I finally tell the clinic, they put me on their mondo anti-itch cream, which helps get me through. I'm still mostly happy to not be in pain or vomiting.

My skin comes off in sheets and chunks, much like the internal tissues. For a time I'm like a zombie. Body pieces are flying off everywhere. Much to my horror, a piece of my heel falls on the bathroom floor after a shower. My heels are not even that dry or cracked, yet there they are, falling off in pieces. Then after a couple of weeks, the process is done. Everything that can come off has come off, like a total body chemical peel.

Gradually, I can do a little more. I'd say it takes about … sixty to ninety days.

Cancer patients are the toughest of the tough. We fight every second of every day. We are not sad or defeated. We know what we've got, and we know what we've gotta do. However, we're not patient. Were it not for the rigid order and logic of our schedules, I can imagine a free-for-all cancer patient stampede at the clinic. Bald heads, wailing and gnashing of teeth, each of us elbowing one another out of the way to be seen first. I regularly see several ladies in the waiting room who could flatten me for sure.

Eventually, I can walk alone safely. I ramp up the housework and start cooking again. I spend more and more time upright and moving instead of sitting. This is a big sign of progress. I'm off IV fluids, have a reduced medication list, and visit the clinic less and less.

But eating remains a struggle. My family gets me exactly what I ask for, and my favorite foods sound great right up until the moment I attempt to eat them. Cajun fried seafood, anchovy pizza, BBQ brisket, Indian, Mexican—I get them all, eat two or three bites, then don't want to even *see* that kind of food for a while. It's disconcerting because I'm used to eating for myself *and* my husband. Now everything tastes like a mixture of cotton and sand.

> Cancer patients are the toughest of the tough. We fight every second of every day. We are not sad or defeated. We know what we've got, and we know what we've gotta do.

One month after my transplant, Dr. Good Ideas thinks I'm doing well. My weight is stable, and I've still only vomited once. I am tolerating my medications and never miss a dose of anything. I have no sign of GVHD. Best of all, I have no cancer symptoms. Every boring, normal lab and exam is a celebration and a victory. Do not miss any visits.

Dr. Good Ideas asks if I'm amazed to not feel my old cancer symptoms. While I'm elated and overjoyed, to be honest, I'm not *amazed*. My unwavering belief was that if I got the transplant, I would live cancer-free. It carried me all along.

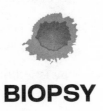

BIOPSY

I've learned to live half alive
Now you want me one more time
Who do you think you are?
Runnin' 'round leaving scars ...
Don't come back for me
Don't come back at all
Who do you think you are?

—CHRISTINA PERRI, "JAR OF HEARTS"

After thirty days, I'm getting my first posttransplant bone marrow biopsy. My resolute expectation is that my graft is thriving and that both my cancers are gone. In all honesty, I expect nothing less. Recalling my first harrowing, tortuous bone marrow biopsy, I opt for sedation this time around. It's a walk in the park, and now I no longer fear them.

A few days later, Dr. Good Ideas calls me in for a special visit to review the biopsy results. Engraftment is perfection. Myelo is gone, no sign of it, and no sign of the chromosomal mutation that caused it. The chemo and the graft took care of it. The ablative chemo ablated, and now the graft is showing up and taking care of business. Myelo, I'm *so* not sad to see you go. This visit is going great!

Then for some reason, Dr. Good Ideas has serious doctor face.

"Your biopsy shows that the Waldenström's lymphoma is still there."

"Still there?"

"Yes. It's still making up around 10 percent of your bone marrow."

I ask Dr. Good Ideas to repeat himself to ensure I heard correctly. Ten percent of my bone marrow is lymphoma. At the time of my diagnosis, it was 40 percent, and just before my transplant, it was 10 to 15 percent. Today's result is minimal change from the pretransplant biopsy. Waldy is still hanging around.

I feel myself diving into the pit of doom. I cannot *believe* Waldy withstood all that chemo. The ablation that almost killed me did not kill my lymphoma. I am clearly dealing with the most chemoresistant, indestructible Keith Richards of cancers. How can this be possible?

I picture Waldy in my marrow weakened, hollow, past his prime, flabby, and out of shape.

"Do you think the lymphoma cells are weakened?"

As usual, Dr. Good Ideas has words of wisdom from the world of science and knowledge. He tells me that yes, the lymphoma cells may be weakened and agrees that yes, they are clearly quite chemoresistant.

"Carol, you need to keep your focus on the mainstay of the treatment: the grafted cells. The graft is therapeutic. Remember, graft versus lymphoma. It's still early, too early to expect complete eradication. I see the graft as the more potent treatment, much more so than chemotherapy. Moreover, we've had to keep the graft's primary mechanism of attacking this lymphoma—the T cells—under control to prevent GVHD. You cannot expect full therapeutic effect yet. It may take twelve to eighteen months, and maybe even up to two years, for the Waldenström's to be gone."

As I take this all in, he continues. "In my opinion, the best news, and the most important consideration, is that you are not experiencing any of your old cancer symptoms. That means more than this biopsy."

I stop myself from snapping back. "Then why did we do the fucking biopsy?"

I didn't say it because I already know the answer: we needed to check on the health of the graft. Dr. Good Ideas seems to be implying that I'm having unrealistic expectations. My sister's overachieving cells should be neutralizing, chomping, and destroying the remaining lymphoma cells, but right now we're holding them back. The graft is not operating at its peak because I am still on immunosuppressive medication. We must wait.

Am I interested in further treatment at this point? Not at all. Not one smidgen. After all, I'm improving. As Dr. Good Ideas so eloquently pointed out, my cancer symptoms are gone.

I have a bad night. I feel like a failure. I don't want to tell anyone; so many people have been through so much. I cannot let them down by *still having cancer*. How can this be possible?

Ultimately, my descent into the pit of doom lasts less than twenty-four hours. Remember, there are no forks in this road. I trust the science and the doctors, and I trust how I feel. I picture Waldy gasping its last breath in my marrow. I must live with him a little longer, but this time it's different because I can't tell he's there.

> I trust the science and the doctors, and I trust how I feel.

Meanwhile, my IgM has had a few blips of elevation but has mostly stayed low. The elevations haven't bothered me too much because as this lymphoma dies, it will release IgM, and it can take a while to clear out. I learned that process. After all, it's a very big molecule.

I try to allow myself to rejoice at the complete eradication of Myelo, as I'd had about one minute to process that wonderful news. I must also rejoice at the health of my graft and the lack of GVHD.

No one ever said my Waldy cure would be immediate. That was all my idea. We couldn't even be sure that my Myelo cure would be so immediate and complete. The Waldy arm of the transplant is more experimental. I know this. Now I'm officially off the ledge, calm, and entertaining the possibility of having reasonable expectations.

DETOURS

Might as well jump
Go ahead and jump
—VAN HALEN, "JUMP"

Around day sixty, I'm feeling perky and optimistic and decide to walk our English cream retriever. I wish I could say he is a good dog; he *tries* to be a good dog, but sometimes he just can't help himself. As we're walking, he pulls me down a hill and then jumps a stream. Before meeting Waldy and Myelo, I could jump across right with him without issue. But today I'm unaware of how weak my muscles are. When I attempt to follow him, I crash knee-first into a rock. My sweet dog runs to me while I'm kneeling in pain. As he sits there whimpering, I can almost hear him say, "Ruh-roh."

I'm a bit embarrassed to confess this little mishap. First, I'm in denial. I get up, walk inside, and take my other dog for a brief, flat walk. *I'm fine,* I think to myself. *A little rest, ice, and elevation and I'll be good to go.* A few hours later, my knee is huge, I cannot walk, and I'm in searing pain.

My seventeen-year-old son is kind enough to drive me to the emergency department of the same hospital in which I had my transplant. To be clear, this does not count as *returning to that hospital*; it's just a visit to the emergency department. The verdict as confirmed by a CT scan: tibial plateau fracture. Fortunately, it's a small fracture line, just a couple of centimeters, and thankfully, it's not displaced. I will not need surgery.

One of the radiology technicians says it best when she comes into my room.

"Oh. *You're* the lady who just had a stem cell transplant and broke her leg walking her dog."

She's laughing.

"Sorry to laugh. Your story is funny."

No worries. We're all laughing. I'm glad I provide some entertainment.

But I'm truly scared to tell Dr. Good Ideas that I broke my leg. After all, I'm supposed to be cautious. When I finally tell him, he is quiet, realizes it's the orthopedic clinic's problem, and moves on. The people in ortho say it will heal well. I have to wear a brace, and they tell me to take it easy. I'm an excellent cancer patient and a horrible ortho patient. My tolerance for compliance and adaptation has been drained. My crutch attitude ranges from poor to tantrum, but fortunately, the fracture heals well.

The lesson here is that feeling stronger and better does not offset muscle weakness. I underestimated my loss of strength, loss of muscle mass, and loss of coordination. Be careful. Do *not* jump the stream.

Around day eighty, I have an intestinal decompensation: hourly explosions, severe cramping, tissue passage, bloating. It persists for a few days, and of course, my thoughts race toward GVHD, which I equate to a death sentence.

I see the cancer clinic physician's assistant. She tells me, "We will treat this as if it's GVHD. Oral steroids, two types. One that stays in the gut, one systemic. We'll start at a very high dose and then wean off over a month if you improve." Lovely. Again, recall that steroids and

I do not get along and that the last time I was on them, I completely lost my mind.

Intestinally—I'm confident that this is a real word—I improve. I have an excellent response to the treatment and am back to normal function within days. Psychologically, I can still feel the irritability, compulsions, and mania creeping up. My options are to sit in a corner rocking and wringing my hands or to get a lot of stuff done quickly. I try to remember that it's the medications.

Dr. Good Ideas suggests a colonoscopy with biopsies to verify GVHD and gauge the severity. Gotta love the endoscopy clinic; they do not mess around. IV in, consent signed, and no memory of anything else. I think they gave me the elephant fentanyl instead of the human fentanyl.

I do not have GVHD. That is correct, young lady, *no GVHD*. Incredible news! The gastroenterologist diagnoses a gastrointestinal infection and secondary inflammation. My poor gut has been through the ringer. I manage to wean off my steroids before I kill anyone.

At ninety days, I can drive, think clearly, and am eating a bit better. I can do some telemedicine appointments, but other than that, I'm not working. I still supervise remotely and still run my business. I'm on strict COVID-19 lockdown, so I do not leave my house except to go to the cancer clinic, which makes my visits quite the social event. I carefully select my leggings and my footwear. Anytime I can get a compliment on my awesome leggings and footwear, I feel great. I do not care if the nurses are humoring me. One nurse likes my snow boots so much that she orders them online from the nurses' station and commands me to look at her computer to verify.

As part of the preventive program, I am referred to the endocrinology clinic. If chemo takes out my thyroid and pancreas but cannot get rid of Waldy, I'm going to be pissed. In the end I check out well for thyroid and don't have diabetes. My bone density scan shows mild low bone density but not osteoporosis. I go on a medication that will prevent further bone loss and potentially even reverse the loss I have.

The endocrinologist says there is a high incidence of gastro-esophageal reflux as a side effect of this new medication. I remind her that my gastrointestinal tract has been torn to shreds by the chemo onslaught and that I just completed an oral steroid course, which has already caused some reflux.

To this she says, "Let's hope for the best and prepare for the worst." I've heard that line before, in *Terms of Endearment*, but lamentably, I let her get away with it. The medication is intolerable. Severe, burning reflux results. Now I know why people with reflux think they're having a heart attack. It ultimately takes me about two months to recover from the reflux. The alternative? An annual IV infusion.

I've been thinking about the varying personalities of the many different clinics I've visited throughout this process. In the blood cancer clinic, everyone's always working. The nurses are all in excellent shape, and they're highly interactive with the patients. They even appreciate cancer humor if you have a good anecdote. They clearly love their jobs.

At the emergency department, they took one look at my oncology alert card, whisked me off to an isolation room, and treated me like royalty. These people do not mess around. They are efficient and quick decision-makers. "Your leg is broken. Here are your instructions and your splint." Then just as quickly as you got in, you're out the door.

Orthopedics has the sketchiest clientele. The characters in that waiting room would make for a great sitcom. The man in line in front of me has no insurance card or driver's license, no paperwork from a referring clinic or physician, and no X-ray reports. When he explains that his driver's license has been suspended, the clerk asks him how he got to the clinic. He drove.

Meanwhile, I'm clutching all of my documents, petrified that they wouldn't see me if I didn't have my things in order. The guy in front of me strolled right on in. The orthopedic receptionist is a saint among humans.

On the other hand, the gastrointestinal endoscopy center handles the entire patient interaction roadblock by opting not to deal with patients at all. They greet me by saying, "Let's put in your IV," then, "You're going to get a little groggy." I must have signed my consent, and I imagine there was a boatload of scopes, pictures, and biopsies, but who knows? I remember only the groggy warning before waking up in the prep area. Barely coherent or able to walk, they tell me I'm ready to go, hand me a packet of photos of the inside of my colon, and throw me into a moving car.

> Maybe one day I'll even hear "normal bone marrow biopsy." That's the dream.

The endocrine clinic may as well be staffed by sloths. No one moves. No one finishes a sentence. The front desk lady walks more slowly than I thought humanly possible.

Oncologists have many euphemisms for when patients are doing reassuringly well: remission, good count(s), excellent engraftment, normal ANC, positive survival rate, stable chemistry, normal physical exam, no GVHD. Lucky patients may even hear "cancer-free." Maybe one day I'll even hear "normal bone marrow biopsy." That's the dream. However, they will not say "cure." Even if you *bribe* them, they will not say cure. It must be the first thing you learn at day one of oncology school. Never say the word "cure" to your patient. At this point I'm considered a "successful transplant." That means I'm not dead yet.

141

APPROACHING SURVIVAL

Share your thoughts, there's nothing you can hide

She was dying to survive

—THE ROLLING STONES, "COMING DOWN AGAIN"

I think of myself as a healthy person. I have a pesky little side item in this whole cancer issue to face, but generally, I'm a healthy person. I tell anyone who will listen that I *will* ride bikes, ski, and climb again. I really want to bag that last fourteener. I want to kayak a class 3 river again. Talking about these physical goals makes them seem real, but I still need a little more strength so I won't break anything, fall off a cliff, or drown. My oldest son thinks he's hilarious when he asks if we should expect a call from the Make a Will Foundation.

Perhaps the best thing about cancer is learning how strong I am. Sometimes, every now and again, I forget I ever had cancer, still *have* cancer, and just had a stem cell transplant. I wake up and feel normal and ready for my day. The pill bottles on the nightstand and my weak limbs soon put me in check, but for occasional, fleeting moments, I manage to forget.

Meanwhile, Dr. Good Ideas does not let me go back to work or to the climbing gym or get on a plane to fly to visit my parents. He grimaces when I tell him I cross-country skied a mile. What could possibly go wrong?

I definitely need a nicer doctor. He is such a royal pain in my ass. He never likes *my* good ideas.

"When can I go swimming?"

"When you are a year out from your transplant," says Dr. Good Ideas.

"May I fly?"

"No."

"May I return to work?"

"No."

"May I climb my last fourteener?"

"Yes. You may do any exercise and physical activity that you feel like doing. You still must stay away from crowds and other potential exposures to sick people. I know you feel great, but your immune system is not yet normal. You are still at risk. It takes time for the grafted cells to produce safe levels of immunoglobulins. We will continue to gradually wean you off of your immunosuppressive medications. We did not do all of this for you to die from a preventable infection."

"Okay."

"Carol, you are doing great. It's wonderful that you feel so well. You must accept a few restrictions for the time being. Now do you have any other unreasonable demands before I leave?"

It's been seven months. I cannot overstate the length of the haul. My biggest challenges remain eating, weakness, and muscle mass. But overall, I feel pretty dang good! The six-to-seven-month range has been a turning point for me. I'm cruising through the potential complications: no broken leg, no diarrhea, no mania, no GVHD. Also, no hair. That will take some time.

I do not think much about the dark days.

While checking in for a respiratory treatment to prevent pneumonia, I see an elderly gentleman in a wheelchair. He's been brushed with the unmistakable cancer colors. Then I recognize two nurses from the bone marrow transplant unit pushing a cart with the initials "BMT" on the side. They ask this gentleman if he's being admitted for a bone marrow transplant, and he says yes. The nurses introduce themselves and load his belongings onto the cart. It feels like yesterday that I was playing out this scene, in this waiting room, on this carpet.

His wife is leaning over, hugging him, sobbing uncontrollably, not wanting to let him go. The nurses reassure her that they will take good care of him. I want to leap up from my chair and tell him how hard this will be but that he will do it and that he will make it. He will go home, get well, and hug his wife again. I want to tell his wife that these nurses will give him the best care he can have anywhere. She will see him again, hopefully in a month. But I cannot say any of this. It would be an invasion of their privacy, and I can't truly promise anything.

I'm sobbing under my mask and wiping my eyes when the respiratory therapist comes to get me. Noticing this, she tells me, "No need to be upset or afraid. This breathing treatment does not hurt." I tell her what's really going on, that I know what he's about to endure. She understands completely.

"You're right. These don't always go well. We see serious complications all the time. But, Carol, you look great! How are you doing?"

"I'm doing great."

At eight months in, I'm approaching normal. My muscles are still weak, but they're getting so much better. I use a rowing machine. I do floor exercises. I skied for two miles on mostly flat terrain and felt great. Weakness is one of the two most significant lingering symptoms, but I feel perceptible strength improvement almost daily and can see my muscles returning.

Food, on the other hand, is still an issue. The crave to aversion cycle is hard to break. Most foods still just taste flat-out bad. Cottage cheese, peanut butter, and most fruits are the lone exceptions. My taste buds are not fully recovered. I still have a stash of barf bags on my nightstand, in the console of my Jeep, in my purse, and throughout the house. I do not know when I will be able to let go of this security blanket.

One of my friends asked for my forgiveness for her not realizing how tough a stem cell transplant is. There's nothing to forgive. Who knew? I myself did not know. My least favorite thing to hear is, "Oh, you poor thing." My favorite thing to hear is, "Your story helped me."

I've had several people ask me how I could possibly have two cancers in my bone marrow. As if I know. None of us gets a free pass. The dice roll, and then they land. Why me? Why not me? I simply must move forward.

Waldy still lives here. I'm not oblivious or in denial that I still have cancer. But in my mind, I'm *well*. Each day that I feel better, my belief in the power of my graft to eradicate

> Cancer immensely sucks, but through it, I learned strength, perseverance, determination, positive outlook, and self-awareness.

Waldy grows stronger. The wonder and awe that I feel toward my new cells does not diminish with time. When I'm sick or need to rest, in illness or recovery, exercise makes me feel worse. When I'm well or getting more energy, exercise makes me feel better.

Time spent fighting cancer and recovering from a transplant is not lost time; it's valuable. This experience has not left me permanently scarred; it has left me permanently *enriched*. Cancer immensely sucks, but through it, I learned strength, perseverance, determination, positive outlook, and self-awareness.

Depending upon my husband to be my caregiver is hard, but I accept it. I let him take care of me. I listen to him. Gradually, I regain my independence. He displays no drama, fear, or bewilderment. He does what he's asked by the cancer clinic staff. He offers me delicate redirection when needed. "I'm glad your stomach is feeling better today, but should you necessarily eat that whole half gallon of ice cream?"

I'm not obligated to speak or otherwise communicate with friends and family every time they reach out. I may be too tired. I may not have clear answers to their questions. I may not be ready to share information. I may feel pressure to always have a positive report or feel guilty sharing negative updates. Constant communication may take up time and energy better spent on resting and self-care. I communicate when I'm ready.

I started feeling sick three years ago and was diagnosed with cancer two and a half years ago. The lag time from symptoms to diagnosis represents my denial period. It took some medical spelunking until I found my way to a hematologist, who diagnosed my cancer after a single visit. Pay attention to your symptoms. Now if I have a question, I ask it. If I have a symptom, I report it. I tell my providers *everything* and follow their instructions.

I received my lifesaving stem cell transplant in the first place because of my diagnosis of Myelo. First, it was a shock, then, in this roundabout way, my savior. In my humble opinion, I believe that physicians and researchers in the field of blood cancer downplay the degree of illness and impairment caused by Waldenström's lymphoma.[2] I continue to believe that stem cell transplants should be more readily considered for Waldenström's lymphoma patients so we can rebrand this disease as *curable*, not merely *treatable*.

No matter how hard you think your stem cell transplant will be, it will be harder. No matter how sick you think you'll feel, you'll feel sicker. And despite that, *it still gets better*.

---

2   I'm a general pediatrician, not an adult oncologist or blood cancer specialist, and I'm only one patient.

BACK TO THE LIVING

Freeze this moment
A little bit longer
Make each sensation
A little bit stronger

—RUSH, "TIME STAND STILL"

Just before my one-year stem cell transplant anniversary, I climbed that last fourteener. It only took fifty-two years from my first—Longs Peak, at age eight—to conquer Culebra Peak at sixty.

It felt great. My husband, middle son, both of my sisters, and two nephews all came along. It was quite a moment, reaching the top. I never knew if I'd live to see it; I never knew if I'd *live* at all. To make it to sixty *and* hike up to this summit fueled by my new cells was more than I could have ever asked for.

My husband buys me a new mountain bike. On our first ride, we ride together for eight miles on an easy, wide, dirt path. *This* is being alive. My goal is to pick up right where I left off and move forward. I cannot let cancer take any more from me.

> My goal is to pick up right where I left off and move forward. I cannot let cancer take any more from me.

At my one-year follow-up bone marrow biopsy, I am hoping for a reduction in lymphoma. By now I fully accept that it may take up to two years for my Waldenström's lymphoma to be completely eradicated. I'm hoping to see a 5–7 percent reading, down from 10 percent. Maybe I'll even be down to 3 percent; *that* would be huge.

After my biopsy, it's Friday, and I'm still waiting for the report. I don't relish having to wait over the weekend to see the results, so I call in to see if someone can snoop it out. Sure enough, a nurse finds it.

"This hasn't been reviewed by your doctor, but it looks good."

I ask if she can send me the full report; I need specifics. She sends it.

I read, "No morphologic or immunohistochemical evidence of lymphoma. Normal bone marrow."

I check to be sure that the report includes my name and birthdate. I check, then double-check, the date of the procedure. I read it over and over. I lie there on the couch and weep with joy. I sob aloud, alone. I have not sobbed like this since the original diagnosis. Then I start jumping up and down. I always believed this would happen, but I did *not* believe it would be this soon. I can't stop rereading the report.

I call my husband and tell him. He's overjoyed. My second phone call is to my donor sister. My blood and marrow studies reveal 100 percent donor cells—all her DNA. There is no evidence whatsoever of my old blood cells. Good job, stem cells.

I reflect on my initial diagnosis, when I was told that I wasn't curable, only treatable, and accepted it. Ha! Wrong! It *is* curable. I'm cancer-free. I'm *cured*.

I recall the exact words my first hematologist spoke to me on the phone as I stood at the gas station in Gunnison. "You have a lymphoproliferative disorder." Now I do not.

I have no disease. The gene that causes the Waldenström's is gone as well. It took three eventful years, with some little ups and downs, but here I am, cancer-free. The release is incredible. The flood of relief and rush of pent-up emotions form a tidal wave of feelings still impossible to label.

I'm ecstatic beyond words with my final result, yet emotionally, over the following couple of weeks, I feel tortured. As the fighting stops, I appreciate everything I've been through. There are so many things I've not allowed myself to feel. I drove by a massive retaining wall after floods and mudslides in Glenwood Canyon and saw them as a stark metaphor of my emotional barricade. One of the cancer clinic nurse practitioners explains that I must process the traumas. There are so many traumas: the diagnosis, the barbaric transplant, the weakness, the process of recovery.

As much as I refuse to let cancer define me, it has become part of my identity. Fighting cancer is a job, a vortex. I still go to the clinic monthly. I have not been on any medication since month eleven. *No* medications. *No* immunosuppressives. I feel wonderful.

I'm plagued with survivor's guilt. I never asked why I had cancer in a philosophical sense. Now I ask why I've survived as others have not. I was otherwise healthy going into the transplant. I can rationalize it, but I still feel guilt at my good fortune. Why me? How am I alive, and why am I cured? Good doctors and good science.

There's also PTSD. I start to recall events in the hospital that I'd forgotten. When I couldn't eat and was vomiting nonstop, I was compelled to ask the nurse when they'd give me total parenteral nutrition to prevent me from starving. He said that it wouldn't be necessary and that I would not starve.

Nevertheless, I pictured myself starving to death in that bed. My nurse knew that I would be able to eat again, but *I* didn't, and I was terrified. I allow myself to relive this, then comfort myself that it didn't come to pass. I am eating, am back to a normal weight, and am nutritionally stable. The nurse was correct—again.

I remember the pain and reexperience it on an even deeper level retrospectively. The clinic staff says that this is all normal and is essential, but I feel stuck in a rerun of the various horrors. Fortunately, this immersion-therapy-like phase passes. I ruminate and emotionally ache until I'm finally set free.

I pull myself out of the hole, settle into reasonable self-expectation, and enjoy the comfort and happiness of being a survivor. I do not want to ever let go of my cancer memories completely. In the end I'm better for it and hope my experience can help others.

I'm finally cleared for part-time work back in my office, and this makes me extremely happy. I receive my COVID-19 vaccines, and they indicate a strong immune response. One of my happiest recovery moments was when I attended an in-person office meeting and got to put on regular clothes. Not baggy sweatpants with a trash bag top but new, matching, bright, stylish, professional clothes. Even without much hair, I suddenly look and feel so human!

Of course, I have physical goals. I want to ski alpine again this winter. I want to work up to riding the Borderline Trail without stopping to rest on the switchbacks. I want to make it to the top without a break. But in the end, I went from pain, sadness, and being bedridden while downing bottles and bags of toxic, lifesaving medication to medication-free, symptom-free, and cancer-free. I learned how to live, mostly happily, through utter physical despair, temporary insanity, and deep uncertainty. I learned how strong I am. I learned that everything can change in an instant and then change back again. It took some time, a few tantrums, and a lot of belief, but it got better.

When I asked my husband to recall his own most intense or meaningful moments in this journey, he mentioned two things. The first was the moment that he picked me up from the hospital. He was so happy to finally see me after that long month. He pictured me as he'd last seen me and pictured me when done with the hardest part. It's human nature: seeing me emaciated and frail was a shock. I had loose skin hanging off bones. He tried to make light of it; he said he felt I had, at best, a fifty-fifty chance of survival. He was shocked to realize that I still might die at home.

His other moment was fascination with the chimerism test, which measures the percent of donor versus recipient cells in the bone marrow and blood. The DNA start point is 100 percent my own, and then with each test posttransplant, there's a higher percent of donor cells and lower percentage of my own, until finally, there's 100 percent donor cells in my bone marrow, blood, and undetectable recipient cells.

In my marrow and blood cells, my sister's DNA is now mine. Now her blood type is also mine. My other bodily cells are still my own DNA, which makes me the proud owner of *two* sets of DNA. I can see a good *CSI* plot coming out of this.

The doctors were not only able to identify the specific genetic mutation that caused my cancers but were also able to get rid of these genetic mutations along with the cancers themselves. That's the most mind-boggling part of all of this for me. My final bone marrow biopsy shows neither of the abnormal genes. I still feel like a character in a sci-fi movie.

Cancer can be beaten. Positives abound, and hope is everywhere in science, treatment advances, outstanding cancer clinics, doctors, nurses, and support groups. I hope that a symptom-free, cancer-free life is also *your* future.

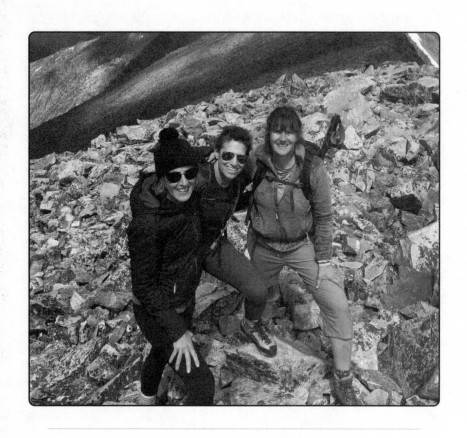

On Culebra Peak, July 2, 2021. I'm in the center with chemo hair.
My older sister, my donor, is to my right, and my younger sister is to my left.

ACKNOWLEDGMENTS

To my husband, Bill Turner, and our three sons, Lander, Dillon, and Conrad Turner, and my two sisters, Donna Rosenwasser and Laura Cornacchione, for their unwavering support.

To my care providers, with special thanks to the nursing staff at the Presbyterian/St. Luke's Medical Center, Denver, Bone Marrow Transplant Unit, for their incomparable expertise.

To my book support team at Advantage Forbes Books for taking a chance on me, with special thanks to Analisa Smith for her beautiful cover design work and to Alec Quig, the absolute best editor on the planet.